The New Prostate Cancer Nutrition Book

The New Prostate Cancer Nutrition Book

by Charles "Snuffy" Myers, MD
Gabrielle Myers
Rose Sgarlat Myers, PT, PhD
Sara L. Sgarlat

Rivanna Health Publications, LLC
Charlottesville, Virginia

TABLE OF CONTENTS

Welcome to this edition of *Eating Your Way to Better Health*, now renamed *The New Prostate Cancer Nutrition Book*. Our first edition was based on my experience with prostate cancer patients and my wife and sister-in-law's Mediterranean family's cuisine. We included many helpful hints and scientific explanations designed to help men who suffer from prostate cancer not only to survive but also to thrive. As the scientific literature on nutrition evolved over the past twelve years, we've learned that the diet we originally recommended, with several modifications for prostate cancer patients, is applicable to people from all walks of life whether they're perfectly healthy or dealing with various diseases. We've also learned that diet is only a part of the equation necessary to staying and becoming healthy after an illness. Exercise, family, friends, hobbies, and relaxation are vital components to a healthy life. For many of us a job or career often substitutes for other aspects of life. Unfortunately for these people, if things go wrong on the job, it is often devastating. We find that this mono-focus on career often leads to unhappiness or depression when one retires because nothing remains to take the job's place, unless one has cultivated other interests.

My (and my co-authors') journeys to develop a lifestyle plan for our family and my prostate cancer patients began with a simple quest for healthful living. At one time, Rose and I were very active in backpacking, hiking, bicycling, canoeing, running, photography, and skiing. We loved the cuisine of Julia Childs and *French Gastronomique*. Red meat, butter, creams and rich desserts were a part of every dinner party we threw in our early adulthood. (Of course, Rose was not raised on this cuisine in her Sicilian parents' household, but my mother embraced traditional American food in all its glory). As we learned about good nutrition from the scientific literature, we dramatically changed our style of eating. And our hobbies changed as our family grew and our professional lives evolved. Rose and I went through periods of less intense structured activity to accommodate our small children. As the children grew, our activity levels with them became more intense.

How Rose and I cooked and ate changed with the times. In the mid 1970s, we gave up butter and rich creams and limited the amount of red meat and other harmful foods we used. We concentrated on low-fat foods, more vegetables, largely white meat, and complex carbohydrates. Several times in the 1980s, we had to promise our overnight babysitters that they could bring their own food to the house lest they go hungry!

First, we concentrated on giving up dairy fat by turning to low or nonfat dairy products and margarine, yet we still consumed some red meat on a weekly basis. My investigations into arachnidonic acid at NIH propelled my reduction of red meat and all dairy fat. Eventually, we found we had to cut red meat from our meals to achieve better health and to help me remain cancer-free. Now, as a rare treat, we enjoy grass-feed red meats two to three times a year.

As our children left home to pursue their independent lives, our activities changed to some degree. Of course, we were also a little older. I became an avid runner once again, albeit somewhat less competitively, and Rose went back to bicycling, but began to cover longer distances. Our adult children enjoy trail running, yoga, and the gym. In the past few years Rose and I have developed a well-equipped exercise room and frequent the athletic club several times a week. We still enjoy hiking, backpacking, kayaking, and skiing, of course. And just like many of my patients and their wives, gardening is a large part of our lives in the Spring, Summer, and Fall. We stay active and spend many hours with family and friends.

Through my personal experiences, my investigations into scientific literature, and the changes I have seen among my own patients and newsletter subscribers, the *Prostate Forum* family (the 'we' of this book) has come to believe that physical activities, social engagements, and relaxing practices can help us retain a positive outlook on life.

We believe that everyone can change when they must. <u>You</u> can change when <u>you</u> must as well. This book will guide you as you move from a traditional American diet and lifestyle to one of optimal health and happiness.

In 1999, when Rose, Sara, and I wrote the first edition of this book, we believed that following a vegetarian diet was the best way to remain healthy and disease-free and so we included many vegetarian and vegan dishes. Well, our opinion changed as the scientific evidence on various diets and foods expanded. We no longer adhere to a vegetarian lifestyle; we now eat a Mediterranean diet of fish, poultry, seafood, and loads of vegetables and fruits. We balance good fats, protein, and carbohydrates in a ratio of 30%, 30%, and 40%. We avoid red meat, dairy fat, and oils and foods rich in omega-6 fatty acids.

You will notice that we added Gabrielle Myers as a new author to this edition. Gabrielle graduated from the California Culinary Academy in 2000. She worked at Oliveto restaurant in Oakland, California for six years, where she learned how to prepare farm-fresh seasonal produce, butcher and cook locally sourced meats, and incorporate health-positive cooking techniques without compromising taste. The vibrant and powerful qualities inherent in each herb, fruit, grain, and vegetable became apparent to Gabrielle in 2006, when she spent the growing season on an organic farm in the Sacramento Valley. For several years, she has honed her cooking skills in restaurants from Virginia to San Francisco. Currently, Gabrielle works as cook and chef for catering companies in Napa Valley and San Francisco. Many of the old recipes written by Rose and Sara now include revised approaches and methods, and Gabrielle and Rose have added new recipes based on the latest scientific research available.

This edition incorporates a decade's worth of new scientific information since we last published. I have incorporated my scientific background with the hands-on knowledge of seeing patients from all walks of life at my clinic, American Diseases for the Prostate (AIDP) (www.prostateteam.com). The diet and other lifestyle suggestions we make are practical and necessary for longevity; our recommendations for cancer patients are also recommended for those with heart problems, cardiovascular diseases, and diabetes. In fact, if you wish to stay healthy or become healthy, you can benefit from the diet and lifestyle plan you'll find in the following pages.

CHAPTER 1

Take Ownership of Your Health

There is a natural tendency for all of us to blindly accept a doctor's advice. The idea is that you have put yourself in the hands of a highly competent professional whom you trust to make appropriate decisions about your health. This is not a good idea. There are many options available in the treatment of prostate cancer and other diseases and no one physician is an expert in the full range of possibilities. There is also a real tendency for physicians to favor the particular approach they use; they are proud of their skills.

But you are a unique patient with unique personal preferences and goals. Two medically equivalent treatments may not be equally beneficial for you. In fact, some patients may prefer a treatment that is less likely to cure them than another simply because they find the side effects of the more aggressive treatment unacceptable. Others are willing to risk any side effect on an untested new treatment for the faintest possibility of a cure. Only you can make these kinds of decisions, not your physician, and only you should develop your own integrated program designed to fight your cancer and to maintain optimal health.

A good way to begin is to reconsider the meaning of health and disease. In medicine, we have long known that health is not just the absence of disease. In truth, most adults who seem healthy actually have several disease processes already underway that they simply don't know about. The young 20-something athlete you see winning a race may already have early stage atherosclerosis. In fact, he may already have cancer! These diseases do not prevent him from being an outward example of vigorous health. This picture of health may continue for many years, or even decades, before the silent disease processes underway finally become apparent. The key point is that happy, healthy, productive people achieve this state of healthiness despite the silent presence of disease. You can be the same way. Just because you have been diagnosed with prostate cancer does not mean that you cannot feel healthy, enjoy your life, and radiate good health. The first step is to take ownership of your cancer and its management. Then you must craft a program that emphasizes health and minimizes disability.

These are the steps in the process of gaining ownership of your health. First, develop an understanding of how health can fail. In collaboration with your physicians, use this information to craft a plan that fits your medical situation and your personal goals. Once this is in place, make certain changes in your life that only you can accomplish. One critical factor is to become physically active. Set up a regular program of exercise designed to promote good balance, strength, and endurance so that you can enjoy life.

You also need to attend to your emotional needs. Studies on happiness repeatedly show that family and friends play a key role in keeping you satisfied and healthy. While having a rewarding job is important, great wealth is less important.

Finally, alter your diet to help you preserve your health. The goal of this book is to explain what we know about diet and health and what you can do about it.

What can you expect if you adopt the dietary recommendations listed in this book? Many patients report to us that they experience an increase in their energy level and feel better than they have in years. The dietary changes we recommend have been shown to help control heart disease, high blood pressure, diabetes, Alzheimer's disease, and several cancers, including colon and prostate cancer. A program of exercise in conjunction with the Mediterranean diet we recommend will also help you fight obesity. These changes are not just for you. In fact, it is hard to change your lifestyle if everyone around you keeps doing the same thing they have always done. Obesity and unhealthy lifestyle choices are contagious. In contrast, families who adopt our recommendations lead healthier, happier lives and each family member finds it easier to make these changes when done together.

CHAPTER 2

Evidence-Based Nutrition

It is very easy to get confused about diet and health. It seems that not a week passes without another report about a new super food. At the same time, we often hear that foods we have always enjoyed are now absolutely lethal. Of course, sometimes these recommendations contradict each other. Some famous dietary gurus recommend a low-fat diet. We also hear that a low carbohydrate diet is the key to staying thin and losing weight. If carbohydrates and fats are bad, that must mean that a high-protein diet is the way to go. But then the *China Study* claimed that high-protein diets cause cancer, heart disease, osteoporosis, and shorten lifespan. If all of this is true and you can't eat protein, fat, or carbohydrates, what's left? Styrofoam and ice cubes are probably not going to make you fat and they are certainly low in cholesterol.

Have you ever tried to figure out which fats are okay? First, we hear that saturated fats are bad. Then we hear that virgin coconut oil is great for your health, but it is one of the most saturated fats available. Then we hear that polyunsaturated fats will lower your cholesterol, but wait—they increase the risk of cancer?

The reason this has become so confusing is that many people who claim to be experts on diet are not very careful about their facts. Many Internet gurus seem to lack any capacity to evaluate evidence and seem to lack even the most basic understanding of biology and yet feel comfortable broadcasting their interpretations to the world.

How can you escape this confusion? In contrast to the dubious information being promoted on some Internet sites, there is a growing body of sound science and clinical investigation that documents a link between diet and the natural history of prostate cancer. Most of this information is contained in papers written by scientists for other scientists in a language with a rather remote relationship to everyday English. Some of the more dramatic results have been mentioned in the media, but a large number of interesting studies remain unnoticed. The goal of this book is to reduce all of this information into an easily adoptable diet and exercise program proven to have a dramatic impact on your health. Since this diet is based on the Mediterranean diet, the cuisine we offer is thousands of years old and remarkably delicious. If you have ever visited an Italian, Greek, Moroccan, or Middle Eastern restaurant, you already have an idea of what the food will taste like. We have also focused on keeping the recipes simple and quick to prepare.

Evidence-Based Nutrition

It is important to understand how we evaluate the scientific literature on the link between diet and health. In general, we should look for dietary items that document a positive impact of diet on the number of deaths attributed to cancer, heart disease and other common illnesses. We should also be looking at the impact of diet on lifespan. The most convincing type of evidence is a clinical trial in which a group of patients are randomly assigned to receive or not receive a component of the diet. These trials typically contain more than 1,000 subjects. The trials must also run for a long enough period of time to gauge the impact of diet, or about 5 to 10 years. We find it more convincing if the design of the trial and its results are also supported by sound laboratory science on the factors governing the growth and spread of prostate cancer. Finally, it is best that any positive trial be run a second time to confirm the result, although this process can easily take 10 to 20 years and millions of dollars to execute.

Large randomized trials are usually preceded by what are called Phase I and II clinical trials. In a Phase I clinical trial, the dose of the drug or nutrient is given in a series of increasing amounts to determine the safest and most effective dose to use for subsequent work. This is followed by a Phase II clinical trial in which a group of patients are treated identically and the impact of treatment determined. This study design is quite common throughout medicine. In fact, a majority of the papers published on the treatment of cancer and heart disease with surgery, radiation therapy, or drugs fit this design.

There are several lines of evidence that are valuable even though they fall somewhat short of this ideal. One common design is to look at a large population and determine which dietary items are more or less common in people who develop various diseases. The best studies of this type ask the patient to identify on an ongoing basis what they are eating and may even involve measuring the levels of a nutrient in the blood or urine. Unfortunately, many studies ask the study participant to remember past dietary patterns. How accurately can you remember how much of which kinds of fat you ate a week ago, let alone over the past five years?

As we discuss each dietary item in this book, we'll mention the evidence that supports its use. In many cases, the evidence is far from complete. Some advocates of evidence-based medicine argue that you should not take any drug if its value has not been proven. We think this strict approach makes little sense when applied to many issues in nutrition. We think a sounder approach is to weigh the potential benefits and risks before making a decision. In several of the cases we'll discuss, the potential benefits are large and the risks nonexistent. The case of cooked tomatoes provides a good example. The proof of their value in the prevention or management of cancer and cardiovascular disease is quite incomplete. Would you stop eating cooked tomato products just because we lack final proof of their value in the management of these diseases? What is the risk to you if you eat cooked tomatoes and subsequent randomized controlled trials show that they really do not prevent prostate cancer, for example? You will still have had the chance to enjoy a good marinara sauce.

The rules we used in designing our dietary recommendations are:

Rule #1: All diseases are not alike.

Leukemias, lymphomas, and cancers of the breast, lung, colon, and prostate are all different diseases. Further, nutritional practices that may be wise for patients with one kind of cancer do not necessarily benefit patients with heart disease. For example, flaxseed oil may lessen the risk of heart disease and may be of value to people with colon or breast cancer, but the scientific evidence we have available today suggests that this oil may <u>increase the risk of metastatic prostate cancer</u>. (For more information on flaxseed oil and prostate cancer, read our booklet *Flaxseed: Panacea or Poison*, available at http://www.prostateforum.com/flaxseed.html). Issues like this have led us to look for specific information on the link between nutrition and the risk of various diseases. Our goal has been to make diet and lifestyle choices that are associated with longevity and that diminish the risk of cancer, heart disease, and other common illnesses.

Rule #2: All dishes must be attractive, tasty, and easy to prepare.

Some of the foods thought to lower the risk of disease include cooked tomatoes, grains, and beans—especially soybeans. Diets that incorporate these elements include the cuisine of the Mediterranean and Asia. Judging from the popularity of Italian, Greek, Japanese, and Chinese restaurants, most Americans find these cuisines appealing. The recipes in this book are drawn largely from the Mediterranean tradition, but also include soybeans and other dietary concepts from Asia.

Rule #3: Judgment is required when information is incomplete or contradictory.

All too often clinical studies on diet and cancer lead to contradictory results. This is particularly the case with dietary fat and health. We have several ways to approach this problem. The first is to recognize that not all clinical studies are of equal quality. We have yet to see a clinical study without some fault. This is so because clinical research is very complex. Some studies have fewer defects or the defects may be relatively unimportant. Second, we are more confident if the results of the clinical trial are consistent with sound laboratory research. A good example of this is the role of antioxidants in health.

CHAPTER 3

Customizing Diet

Have you noticed there is a diet for every persuasion? And it seems as if you can find an Internet site that claims to medically justify any diet you want. For each of these diets one can present a scientific or pseudoscientific rationale. These sites usually also give case histories or testimonies of people who have had success with the diet in question. This is can be very confusing. If all these diets work, does it mean that eating anything will work?!

Some commonly advocated diets are:

Vegan Diet:
  high carbohydrate, low fat, and rich in grains and legumes
Atkins and South Beach Diets:
  high protein, high fat, and low carbohydrate
Paleolithic Diet:
  high in wild meat, root vegetables, and nuts but no grains or legumes
Zone Diet:
  30/30/40 balance of protein, fat, and carbohydrate
Mediterranean Diet:
  low in animal products, low in protein, rich in grains and legumes, and rich in monounsaturated and omega-3 fats
Chinese Diet:
  low in animal products, low in protein, and rich in plant products
Okinawan Diet:
  favors modest calorie restriction and relies on tofu and fish as major protein sources
Low-Glycemic Carbohydrate Diet:
  only low-glycemic carbs

We think this confusion partly results from bad science. It is also true that people differ significantly in how their bodies respond to various dietary changes. The best diet for you will depend on your genetics. This is a hot new area of nutritional research, but the evidence supporting the approach is quite old.

Between 1999 and 2000, Professor Tim Noake's group at the University of Cape Town took an important step toward measuring this variability. They studied a group of 61 trained cyclists. After an overnight fast, they measured the percent of energy derived from burning fat versus carbohydrate. At rest, the proportion using fat ranged from a low of 25% to a high of 100%. When these cyclists were exercised at 70% of their maximum heart rate, fat contributed anywhere from 0 to 40%. Think about these results: some people are readily able to switch to fat burning for all their energy at rest and up to 40% at a relatively intense level of exercise, while others appear to have great difficultly switching to fat burning even when at rest. Now, you can see how people who burn fat well can lead a normal life and feel fine on a high protein/high fat diet, while those who need carbohydrate just feel terrible. So, one area in which we differ is that some of us are fat-burners and others carbohydrate-burners, but most of us are a mixture of these two extremes.

There are similar differences in how well people tolerate high carbohydrate diets. Some will rapidly gain abdominal fat, experience an increase in serum triglyceride levels, and a dramatic decline in their good (HDL) cholesterol. Others seem to thrive on a high carbohydrate diet.

We think it has long been apparent that diets need to be tailored to the individual, at least so far as the amount of fat versus the amount of carbohydrate goes. One simple approach is to look for evidence of carbohydrate excess in their diet. This approach starts with the lipid panel that family doctors get on most adults to screen for high cholesterol. This test reports the total cholesterol, the bad or LDL cholesterol, the good or HDL cholesterol, and the triglycerides. If you eat too many carbohydrates, your triglycerides will tend to increase and your good or HDL cholesterol will tend to fall. A relatively simple measure is to look at the ratio of the serum triglyceride divided by the HDL cholesterol. Under optimal conditions, this will approach 1.0. In patients approaching diabetes mellitus, the ratio can reach 7 or 8. An elevated ratio indicates you are probably taking in more carbohydrate than you can safely handle. We will return to this later in the book when we talk about meal planning.

We are soon to witness a revolution in the area of personal diet design. Scientists are already identifying the key genes involved in your dietary interactions. While our knowledge is still incomplete, clinical trials testing gene analysis to tailor diets are being published. This field now even has a name, nutrigenomics. A clinical trial recently published in the *Nutritional Journal* by Arkadianos, et al. (*Nutrition Journal* 2007, 6:29) can give you insight into this new field. This article is available to you in its entirety via the web as part of the Creative Commons Attribution License. In this study, they screened for variations in 19 genes involved with nutrition. They then designed a diet for each patient based on their gene profile. The group on the nutrigenomics diet lost 4.2 pounds compared with a 1.2-pound gain in the others. There was also a significant reduction in serum blood sugars on the custom tailored diet. This is clearly a very rapidly moving area with great promise.

In the next edition of this book, we may well be talking about how to use your nutrigenomics result, but for now, we will be limiting ourselves to your triglyceride/HDL ratio.

Hunter-Gatherer Versus Farmer

How can it be that humans exhibit such dramatic genetic variation in how they interact with food? The most likely explanation is that this reflects the history of our species. It is important to delve into this issue so that you can later understand why certain aspects of diet are so important. This means delving in some detail into human evolution—as it is important for you to understand how humans ended up being the way we are.

Humans share a close kinship with the other great apes, such as the species of chimpanzees, gorillas, and orangutans. If you go to the zoo and look at the other members of this group, the physical resemblance is clear. There are obvious differences that separate us from the other great apes beyond our intellectual accomplishments. We stand upright and are relatively hairless. When we move, the differences become dramatic. None of the other great apes walk with the ease and efficiency that we do. However, the real differences come when we start to run. It is really revealing to watch children run. Somewhere between ages 3-4, they just seem to discover how to run with a fluid motion.

If you want to understand in greater detail how humans are adapted to running and the implications of this adaptation, I recommend you read Christopher McDougal's recent book *Born to Run*. This book provides a detailed review of how humans are adapted to run. It even provides a colorful account of a hunter-gatherer group running game into the ground.

These differences are critical to understanding how we've evolved and our nutritional requirements.

A recent series of papers has served to emphasize the anatomy that supports this fluid running style. The human foot has an arch and spanning this arch is a broad tendon called the plantar fascia that starts at the base of the toes and attaches to the front of the heel. At the back of the heel, the Achilles tendon attaches and passes up to the muscles of the calf. During running, this combination of plantar fascia and Achilles tendon act as a spring that is stretched as the foot is planted and then rebounds as the foot leaves the ground. This elastic recoil makes the human running stride remarkably efficient: up to 50% of the energy involved in running comes from this elastic recoil. While humans are far from the fastest runners, we are one of the most efficient in terms of the energy cost of covering ground.

A second major innovation is the nature of the human skull. The human skull is very efficient at disposing heat to keep the brain cool. The fact that we are largely hairless and sweat so well adds to our ability to withstand heat. The combination of our efficient running style and our ability to tolerate heat means that human hunters can run most prey to exhaustion even in the middle of a hot day. A current belief is that humans arose as endurance predators and scavengers.

This capacity to cover ground easily apparently developed before we were fully human: Homo erectus had a foot identical to ours and was built for running. However, the Homo erectus brain was much less well developed. The point is that the hunting lifestyle is very old and human adaptation to that lifestyle quite apparent. Human remains dating from before the great Ice Age revealed people who were tall and well-nourished. The hunter-gatherer lifestyle was already well established.

Recent detailed reviews of the hunter-gatherer lifestyle that incorporate what we know of existing groups as well as the fossilized remains, paint an interesting picture. Of those who survived to age 15, approximately two thirds reached age 70. Approximately 70% of the deaths came from infections, with cardiovascular disease and cancer being relatively uncommon. More than half the calories came from animal products, but these are of a much broader range than we use now. Small game (rabbits, birds, rodents), insects, fish, and other marine organisms were widely used. The plant foods tended to be dominated by greens, nuts, and root vegetables. Grains and legumes were not common food items. This diet was rich in protein and fat and often limited in carbohydrate. In this setting, it is of advantage to be able to burn fat as an energy source.

As these discoveries have come to light, some have focused on this as a rationale to make red meat a health food. However, commercially available red meat differs chemically in important ways from what is found in wild game. Corn and other common grains used to feed ruminants are rich in omega-6 fatty acids and poor in omega-3 fatty acids. Because the balance between these two fats is so important, foods are ranked by the amount of omega-6 as compared to the amount of omega-3 fats. Dividing the omega-6 content by the omega-3 content easily does this. Red meat at your grocery store may have a ratio of omega-6 to omega-3 in the 6-7 range. In wild game, the ratio is closer to 1. Corn has an omega-6 to omega-3 ratio of 40-50, so a little bit of corn in the diet can really change the ratio quite dramatically.

Of course, the hunter-gatherer lifestyle is also a very active one. They did not need the equivalent of a health club to keep in shape: the daily effort to stay alive and well-fed did not allow for sloth.

One key limitation to the hunter-gatherer lifestyle is that most environments only support limited populations; food was not dependable, and periodically there would not be enough food.

The next big step was the development of agriculture. Grains and legumes offer abundant yields from limited land. Fewer acres can provide enough calories for a family, and grains and legumes can be stored to provide food when game might not be available. However, grains and legumes are mostly carbohydrate with protein contents that range from 10-20%; in addition, these food sources are low in fat. Suddenly, the survival diet is high carbohydrate and low in protein and fat.

This is not a diet to which humans were well adapted. Skeletal remains dating from the transition to agriculture do not paint the same picture of robust, vigorous health seen in hunter-gatherer societies. However, you could feed more people and limit the risk of starvation, so human populations exploded with the development of agriculture.

Those who adapted to the farming diet had a survival advantage. Agriculture arose in the Fertile Crescent and extended to Europe and India. Today, most of the people who live around the Mediterranean and throughout Europe speak languages that trace back to those early farmers: they bear the genes of those farmers as well. This dramatically illustrates the survival advantage provided by farming: the offspring of farmers dominate the populations of Asia, India, the Mediterranean Basin, and Northern Europe.

While agriculture appeared about only 10,000 years ago, our genes show evidence of adaptation to the farming lifestyle. Wheat, rye, and barley all contain gluten and those who can tolerate gluten can access the nutrition in the grain. This adaptation is now dominant throughout the Middle East and Europe. Gluten tolerance was a genetic adaptation to farming.

The ability to tolerate lactose, the sugar in milk, is also a recent evolutionary change. In most hunter-gatherers, the capacity to digest milk sugar is lost in adult life. In the farming populations of Europe, the ability to digest milk sugar persists in adult life. Populations with this genetic change can use milk and milk products for protein and fat as adults. Dairy farming can successfully use farmland for other crops and this can provide an important survival advantage.

Amylase is an enzyme in saliva needed to break down the carbohydrates in grains. Those descendants of farmers now bear multiple copies of the amylase gene. People with this genetic change can more easily digest grains, again providing a survival advantage.

It is quite likely that the shift to tolerating high carbohydrate diets and burning carbohydrate instead of fat represents an evolutionary adaptation to farming. Carbohydrate is a very high-octane fuel. During exercise, you can generate much more energy per minute using carbohydrate than you can using fat. If carbohydrates were available and tolerated, there would be a considerable survival advantage in being able to use that effectively. Today, runners from Kenya and Ethiopia dominate track events, from the mile to the marathon. Both of these populations are traditional subsistence farmers who survive on a diet composed largely of grains and legumes where protein and fat are much lower than in the typical hunter-gatherer diet.

Humans today reflect this complex history. We see it in the way we vary in our abilities to use carbohydrate versus fat as fuel. We also see this evolutionary history in the way we vary in our responses to calorie excess and calorie restriction. Your search for a diet that matches your genetics will be easier if you take these issues into consideration. We have written this book with this in mind. You will be able to select recipes that vary in carbohydrate, fat, and protein content according to your individual physiology. Overall, we recommend a balance of protein, carbohydrates, and fats in a 30%, 40%, 30% ratio.

Here are some ideal ranges for your lipid panel, blood pressure and blood sugar.

LDL cholesterol	Less than 100
HDL cholesterol	More than 50
Triglycerides/HDL cholesterol	1-2
Systolic blood pressure	Under 120 mmHg
Fasting blood sugar	Less than 90

If your numbers are not ideal, you should first try to adjust your diet and lifestyle. The rest of this book is designed to help you reach these goals. It is our opinion that drugs should only be used if you cannot reach these goals on your own.

How can you adjust your diet to fit your needs? Today, the simplest approach is to look at your lipid panel. Carbohydrate intake in excess of your needs will tend to increase the triglycerides and decrease the HDL cholesterol. If you divide the triglycerides by the HDL cholesterol, the ratio should be under 2. If it is above 5, you are in trouble and need to make a major change in your lifestyle. If it is above this, it is likely that you are eating too much carbohydrate compared with heart-healthy fat and protein.

You can improve this by decreasing the amount of carbohydrate you eat in each meal and making sure that you are eating appropriate amounts of fat and protein. The remainder of this book will help you reach this goal.

CHAPTER 4

Salt

For over 50 years, people have been encouraged to lower their salt intake, yet it appears that during that time salt intake in the United States has remained constant at 3.7 grams a day. In one recent review of salt intake from 33 countries in studies involving close to 20,000, participants showed a relatively narrow range of 2.7 to 4.9 grams a day. To put this in perspective, one teaspoon is roughly 2.5 grams. It is really quite remarkable that the intake of salt remains so relatively constant across different cultures. This has led investigators to propose that there is a strong biological regulation of salt intake. The implication of this idea is that humans will reliably avoid both very high and very low salt intake without conscious effort.

In fact, human history clearly establishes that humans have a natural drive for salt consumption. Some of the earliest examples of trade involve salt. (Interestingly, the word salary comes from the salt ration used as payment to the soldiers of Rome.)

How do the current recommendations for salt intake compare with what people seem to do naturally? In the United States, the recommended intake is 2.3 grams. Those with chronic renal disease or at risk for hypertension are told to limit their intake to 1.5 grams. Those who exercise vigorously are allowed 3 grams a day. These risk factors include being African-American, being over 40, having a systolic blood pressure above 120 mmHg, or having a diastolic blood pressure above 80 mmHg. Unfortunately, a very large portion of the American population fits those definitions. It is also unfortunate that people do find it very difficult to stay on a low salt diet, but this should not be a surprise given the evidence that humans naturally gravitate toward a 2.7-4.9 gram a day intake.

In contrast to this set of observations, many clinical and population studies point to a large benefit to reducing salt intake. One recent influential review estimated reducing salt intake by 3 grams per day would reduce deaths by 44,000 to 92,000. Keep in mind that prostate cancer deaths are between 20-30,000, so this number is quite significant. The estimated reduction in health care costs annually would run 10-24 billion dollars.

If people cannot be depended on to voluntarily reduce their salt intake, what are the options? The potential benefit in lives and money saved have fueled an effort to pressure the food and restaurant industries to reduce the salt content of food in the United States. In simple terms, if people will not do this voluntarily, then we will create a situation in which virtue is forced on them. I could be wrong about this, but government regulation has a poor track record of controlling human biologic drives. For this to work, saltshakers would have to be taken off the tables at restaurants. At home, people would just add salt until the food tasted right to them.

How do we come to regulate our salt intake? When your blood volume, blood pressure or sodium concentration of your blood drops, your kidneys release the hormone renin. Renin then results in the production of angiotensin I, which is converted to angiotensin II. The latter causes blood vessels to constrict, increasing your blood pressure. It also causes the production of aldosterone, a hormone that causes the kidneys to decrease the amount of salt lost in the urine. Aldosterone also works on a part of the brain, called the amygdyala, to cause salt hunger in animals. Thus, if salt intake drops below your body's set point, it will actively try to stop salt loss and cause you to crave salt.

The increase in angiotensin triggered by a low salt diet can have other detrimental actions. In addition to this physiologic role, abnormal activation of the renin angiotensin system plays an important role in hypertension. Drugs that block this pathway are among the agents most effective in the treatment of hypertension. Angiotensin II is also involved in congestive heart failure, atrial fibrillation, the development of diabetes, and the termination of penile erections. Finally, angiotensin II has been described as one mechanism of hormone resistance in prostate cancer. I think it is not an accident that in some clinical trials a very low salt diet actually proved detrimental.

In the face of these disturbing issues, we have elected not to focus on low salt recipes. If your doctor recommends a low salt diet, it is easy enough for you to eliminate or reduce the salt in any given recipe. For soups and stews, some added lemon juice can reduce the need for salt.

CHAPTER 5

Antioxidants & Prostate Cancer

There is quite an extensive scientific literature on antioxidants and prostate cancer. It is an area of great interest to patients and, at the same time, one of great confusion. The whole role of antioxidants in prostate cancer prevention and treatment has become quite controversial because of conflicting studies. As this edition goes to print, these controversies are far from settled.

What causes oxidative damage to prostate tissue? In a series of laboratory studies, George Wilding, MD and his colleagues (Ripple, et al.) at the University of Wisconsin have shown that adding testosterone to human prostate cells causes the release of strong oxidants that can damage these cells. The addition of the antioxidants selenium, vitamin E, or vitamin C lessens the oxidative damage caused by testosterone. While this might make the intake of antioxidants like selenium and vitamin E seem wise, we will learn that these antioxidants also cause serious side effects. We will demonstrate that it is best, for the most part, to obtain your antioxidants from food rather than from pills.

Common antioxidants include:

Vitamin E
Selenium
Vitamin C
Lycopene (Tomatoes, watermelon, red grapefruit)
Polyphenols (Green tea, chocolate, grapes)
Anthocyanins (Red/purple fruits and vegetables)
N-Acetylcysteine (NAc)

Mitochondria convert food into an energy form that cells can use. Ripple, et al. have shown that testosterone-induced oxidant formation is associated with major alterations in the mitochondria, and it seems likely that the mitochondria are the cell site where these oxidants are generated. I should point out that the observations by Ripple, et al. have been confirmed in such a way that I have no doubt that this is occurring. This would not be unusual, because there are many other situations in which the mitochondria have been shown to be the major sites of oxidant generation.

The major limitation to Dr. Wilding's studies is his laboratory setting. Laboratory findings such as these need to be extended to studies on human prostate tissue obtained during radical prostatectomy or during an autopsy. Such an analysis has been done in a very innovative fashion. Damage to the DNA, the genetic material in a cell, can lead to cancer. Strong oxidants are just one of a number of mechanisms through which such DNA damage occurs. Fortunately, oxidative damage to the DNA results from chemical alterations in the DNA that cannot be the result of any other process. Malins and colleagues have examined DNA from the prostates of men with and without cancer. They showed that the amount of oxidative damage to prostate DNA increased steadily with age. They also looked at whether the extent of oxidative damage to DNA correlated with the development of prostate cancer. At low levels of oxidative DNA damage, there was no correlation with prostate cancer. However, above a certain level, the risk of cancer increased dramatically with escalating DNA damage until the risk exceeded 90%! These results fit beautifully into the natural history of prostate cancer and offer an explanation of why prostate cancer is a disease that usually occurs in men over the age of fifty; it takes decades to accumulate enough DNA damage to cause cancer.

Dr. L. Clark, from the University of Arizona, randomized more than one thousand healthy subjects to one of two groups: one took selenium-yeast and one did not. After ten years, the approximate reduction in overall cancer deaths in the group on selenium was 50%. Prostate cancer was the malignancy most affected with a greater than 60% reduction in death rates. In this trial, no side effects were observed when researchers administered a dose of 200 micrograms of selenium. In my opinion, the safety of this dose has now been abundantly confirmed by other studies. These results were impressive, because this dose of selenium caused only a doubling of the serum selenium levels. The results of Dr. Clark's study have been supported by a number of non-randomized clinical studies, confirming that men with higher blood or nail selenium levels have a reduced risk of developing and dying from prostate cancer.

Now, this result has become controversial. A subsequent randomized controlled trial failed to show any benefit to selenium in prostate cancer prevention. Unfortunately, the new clinical trial used selenomethionine and not the selenium-yeast used in the Clark trial. So, did this new trial fail because they used the wrong form of selenium?

Finnish investigators designed a clinical trial to test whether vitamin E or beta-carotene would alter the risk of lung cancer in cigarette smokers. Close to 23,000 subjects were divided into four groups: One received no treatment. The remaining three were given beta-carotene alone, vitamin E alone, or beta-carotene plus vitamin E. When the trial had been running between 5 and 8 years, investigators noted that men on vitamin E alone had a 34% reduction in the risk of developing prostate cancer. The group also experienced a 40% reduction in prostate cancer death rates compared to the "no treatment" group. In contrast, taking beta-carotene alone was associated with an increase in prostate cancer deaths, while the "vitamin E plus beta-carotene" group had results similar to the "no treatment" group.

There are a number of factors that make the results of this trial surprising: First, the dose of vitamin E (50 International Units) is much lower than the doses commonly found in health food stores (between 200 and 1,000 International Units) and thought to be quite safe. Second, the vitamin E used in the trial was produced artificially rather than naturally. Consequently, it had only half the activity of the naturally-occurring form. Third, the alpha form was used, which is much less active than the gamma or delta form of this vitamin. In other words, the investigators' choice of vitamin E dose and form minimized any potential benefit. In view of these issues, it is truly amazing that they observed a 40% death rate reduction in the arm of the study receiving vitamin E alone.

Again, a subsequent randomized controlled trial failed to show any impact of vitamin E on the incidence of prostate cancer. The form of vitamin E used in this new trial was alpha tocopherol, the same form used in the earlier Finnish study. However, laboratory studies had shown that alpha tocopherol was the least active form of vitamin E. Gamma tocopherol and gamma tocotrienol were the most active. In fact, one recent interesting laboratory paper showed that tocotrienol would arrest growth of prostate cancer stem cells. Would vitamin E have proved active if one of the more active forms had been used? I fear we may never know.

There is a third, small clinical trial that tested the impact of lycopene, the red pigment in tomatoes. Lycopene is a relative of beta-carotene that differs in two ways. First, lycopene is a much more effective antioxidant than beta-carotene. Second, beta-carotene can be converted to vitamin A, but lycopene cannot. In the clinical trial (Kucuk, et al.), twenty-six men were randomized to receive nothing or 15 mg of lycopene twice a day for three weeks before radical prostatectomy. Among the men on lycopene, 73% showed surgical margins free of cancer or no evidence of spread beyond the prostate gland compared to 18% in the "no lycopene" group. There was also a statistically significant reduction in the presence of high-grade prostatic intraepithelial neoplasia (a premalignant lesion of the prostate) in the men on lycopene.

The most provocative aspect of Kucuk's lycopene trial was a significant decline in IGF-1 blood levels. IGF-1 is a major growth and survival factor for prostate cancer cells. Elevated IGF-1 blood levels are associated with an increased risk of prostate cancer. Additionally, the changes that IGF-1 causes in prostate cancer cells are commonly enhanced by the development of hormone-resistant prostate cancer. The second provocative aspect of this trial concerns the radical prostatectomy specimens. Analysis suggests that lycopene may cause cancer regression, which implies that it can also cause cancer cell death. As we will see later, other antioxidants appear to be able to kill prostate cancer cells. This small trial is noteworthy but needs to be confirmed.

Again, a subsequent large randomized controlled trial failed to show any impact of lycopene on the incidence of prostate cancer. While this clinical trial was being conducted, laboratory studies showed that lycopene itself had no activity against prostate cancer, but that some related carotinoids in the tomato extract did. The next step would be to look at the clinical activity of these related carotinoids.

While these trials were taking place, research on the genetic basis of prostate cancer was proceeding. Several studies found an enzyme, Mn-superoxide dismutase (MnSOD), existed in a mutated form that appeared to be associated with an increased risk of prostate cancer. This was interesting because MnSOD acts to protect mitochondria, the energy plant of the body, from oxidative damage. Prostate cancer cells are rich in mitochondria and this is the site where Ripple, et al. documented testosterone-induced oxidation. There were then studies to show that men with the mutated form of MnSOD were more likely to experience a large drop in the risk of prostate cancer if they consumed antioxidants. Unfortunately, there then followed a sequence of studies that failed to document any convincing link between MnSOD, prostate cancer, and benefits from antioxidants.

Plants contain a range of compounds called polyphenols. Many of these are powerful antioxidants. The health benefits of green tea, cocoa, red wine, pomegranate, blueberry and a range of other fruits are thought to arise from their polyphenol content. As we write this chapter, a large randomized controlled trial is testing the benefit of one of these: pomegranate. We will not venture a guess if this trial will be positive or not, but we will cover in greater detail the existing literature on pomegranate in the next section.

We think it is important to note that all of the antioxidants tested, especially the polyphenols and carotinoids, have other effects that have nothing to do with the fact that they are antioxidants. It may well be that each of the compounds that exhibit anticancer activity do so independently of the fact that they are antioxidants. Perhaps antioxidant activity is a red herring and we need to be looking elsewhere. At the very least, no one should choose a food item because some lab test shows it has the most antioxidant activity. I can find no clinical association between laboratory tests of antioxidant activity and clinical benefit.

We recommend a Mediterranean diet. It also happens to be rich in antioxidants because it is rich in fruits and vegetables, but the antioxidant content is not the reason to adopt this diet. We do so because there are multiple randomized controlled trials documenting a benefit from this diet. This literature is reviewed in the next chapter.

Anthocyanins (Red/Purple Fruits)

Eating red/purple fruits such as grapes, raspberries, strawberries and pomegranates is associated with multiple health benefits. These fruits and their juices are very rich in antioxidant activity. While much is made of this fact in the media and in marketing materials, the health benefits of these foods likely has a much more complex basis. These issues have been most completely investigated for pomegranates and so we will review this story in some detail. Ahead of time, we would note that blackberries, blueberries, and black raspberries may well have similar benefits.

Currently, interest in pomegranate is based on the prostate cancer clinical trial by Pantuck. The pomegranate juice used was that marketed by the POM Wonderful Company. In the first step in this trial, the authors looked at serum antioxidant activity after doses of juice of 0, 3, 6, 9, 12 and 15 oz a day. The serum antioxidant activity increased steadily with dose. The conclusion of this initial test was that a dose of 6-8 oz would give considerable serum antioxidant activity, but not deliver too much sugar to increase blood sugar or serum triglycerides. They chose 8 oz a day as the dose. This is obviously a fairly arbitrary way to choose the dose. It would have been much better to do a dose-finding study, which looked at the impact of various doses on anticancer activity rather than antioxidant activity.

The second step was a Phase II clinical trial. In Phase II clinical trials, all patients are treated with what is thought to be the optimal treatment and the response measured. This was not a randomized comparison. 48 patients entered the study, but only 46 participated fully. All 46 had failed initial treatment for prostate cancer, including radical prostatectomy or radiation therapy. The Gleason scores ranged from 5-7, so this was a study of intermediate grade cancers, not aggressive high-grade disease (Gleason 8-10). While 63% were organ-confined, 37% had locally advanced cancer that had spread outside the prostate capsule or invaded into the seminal vesicles. At the time they entered the study, the median PSA was 1.05 ng/ml, so this was relatively early in the development of their metastatic disease. For each patient, the PSA doubling time was measured before study entry with a minimum of three determinations over a period of 6 months. Once on the study, PSA levels were determined every 3 months.

The patients were treated in two stages. In the first stage, 24 patients were treated and four had greater than a 50% decline in PSA. At this point, the trial was extended to accrue the final 46 patients. The goal of the paper was to measure the ability of this juice to slow the rate of cancer growth, which required the comparison of the PSA doubling time before and after starting treatment. One problem the investigators encountered was that at 24 months, 7 out of 46 patients had a negative PSA doubling time. In other words, their PSAs were declining rather than increasing. For this reason, the duration of the clinical trial was extended beyond the planned 24 months. At 33 months, 3 of the 7 had now developed an increasing PSA.

At 33 months, the average pretreatment PSA doubling time was 15.6 months compared with 54.7 months after treatment. During the study, 83% of the patients experienced an improvement in their PSA doubling time. The impact of the treatment was highly significant statistically with a P less than 0.0001. No side effects were noted and no patient developed detectable metastatic disease during the trial.

Because pomegranate juice contains compounds that have phytoestrogen activity, they examined the impact on hormone levels. There was no significant change in testosterone, estradiol, sex hormone-binding globulin, IGF-1, DHEA, or androstenedione.

Pomegranate fruit extracts are available that concentrate on one component, ellagic acid. However, this fruit is a complex mixture of chemicals other than ellagic acid that have important health benefits. These compounds are found in the juice-containing capsules, seeds (punicic acid), peel and even the flower. At this point, all of the investigators who have examined the activity of these chemicals have found that the combination is more effective than any single individual component. There are now capsules available that contain extracts of the juice alone or a combination of the various parts of the fruit. These capsules have two advantages over the fruit and the juice: less sugar and easier to take on trips.

Chemicals found in pomegranate include:

Ellagic acid and polymers of this polyphenol (punicalagin)
Caffeic acid
Luteolin
Punicic acid
Anthocyanin pigments, particularly delphinidin

There is also some evidence that pomegranate may improve cardiovascular health and we have included citation to papers on that subject, listed below.

References On Oxidative Damage:

M. Ripple, et al. "Prooxidant-antioxidant shift induced by androgen treatment of human prostate carcinoma cells" *Journal National Cancer Institute* 89: 40, 1997.

M. Ripple, et al. "Androgen-induced oxidative stress in human LNCaP prostate cancer cells is associated with multiple mitochondrial modifications" *Antioxid Redox Signal* 1: 71, 1999.

M. Ripple, et al. "Effect of antioxidants on androgen-induced AP-1 and NF- kappaB DNA- binding activity in prostate carcinoma" *Journal National Cancer Institute* 91: 1227, 1999.

P.H. Gann, et al. "Lower prostate cancer risk in men with elevated plasma lycopene levels: results of a prospective analysis" *Cancer Research* 59: 1225, 1999.

O.P Heinonen, et al. "Prostate cancer and supplementation with alpha-tocopherol and beta-carotene: incidence and mortality in a controlled trial" *Journal National Cancer Institute* 90: 440, 1998.

L. C. Clark, et al. "Effects of selenium supplementation for cancer prevention in patients with carcinoma of the skin. A randomized controlled trial. Nutritional Prevention of Cancer Study" *Journal American Medical Association* 275: 1957, 1996.

L. C. Clark, et al. "Decreased incidence of prostate cancer with selenium sup- plementation: results of a double-blind cancer prevention trial" *British Journal Urology* 81: 730, 1998.

O. Kucuk, et al. "Phase II randomized clinical trial of lycopene supplementation before radical prostatectomy" *Cancer Epidemiol Biomarkers Prev* 10: 861, 2001.

L. Chen, et al. "Oxidative DNA damage in prostate cancer patients consuming tomato sauce-based entrees as a whole-food intervention" *Journal National Cancer Institute* 93: 1872, 2001.

D.C. Malins, et al. "Age-related radical-induced DNA damage is linked to prostate cancer" *Cancer Research* 61: 6025, 2001.

References On Pomegranate:

Pantuck, AJ, et al. "Cancer Therapy: Clinical Phase II Study of pomegranate juice for men with rising prostate-specific antigen following surgery or radiation for prostate cancer". *Clinical Cancer Research* 12: 4018-26, 2006

Aviram, M, et al "Pomegranate juice consumption for 3 years by patients with carotid artery stenosis reduces common carotid intima-media thickness, blood pressure and LDL oxidation". *Clin Nutr* 23: 423-33, 2004

Sumner, MD et al. "Effects of pomegranate juice consumption on myocardial perfusion in patients with coronary artery disease" *Am J Cardiology* 96: 810-4, 2005.

CHAPTER 6
Omega-3 Fatty Acids

We now know that certain fats are essential for optimal health and even for survival. These essential fats are divided into two groups: omega-3 and omega-6 fats. We find omega-6 in poultry and meat, egg yolks, and most vegetable oils. Omega-3 fatty acids occur in fish as well as in some nuts, seeds, and their oils. Contemporary American and Northern European diets are very rich in omega-6 fats and it's virtually impossible for most of us to develop a deficiency. One reason for this is that corn is the major feedstock for agriculture and it is very rich in omega-6 fatty acids. On the other hand, omega-3 deficiency is quite common.

Let's look a little more closely at the omega-3 fatty acid found in flaxseed, because its role as a source of omega-3s is widely touted today.

There are three common omega-3 fatty acids found in our diet. ALA is the smallest and is a chain of 18 carbons in a row. ALA can be converted to EPA, which is 20 carbons long. Finally, EPA can be converted into DHA, which is 22 carbons long. It is EPA and DHA that are essential for human health.

As we just mentioned, omega-3 fats occur in marine fish as well as in certain nuts, seeds, and oils. Alpha-linolenic acid (ALA) is the omega-3 fatty acid found in flaxseed. EPA and DHA, on the other hand, are the omega-3 fats found in ocean fish. The fish do not make EPA and DHA, but obtain it from the algae that are at the bottom of the ocean food chain. In the algae, EPA and DHA act to keep their cell membranes functioning at cold temperatures. Thus, fish who live in cold waters tend to have the greatest EPA and DHA content.

ALA is much less active than DHA and EPA and its health benefits are largely limited to cardiovascular health. But even for cardiovascular disease, ALA is less effective than EPA and DHA. But, it's not that simple because, to some extent, your body converts ALA into EPA and DHA. And nutritionists and alternative health experts use this fact as the scientific justification to market oils and foods rich in ALA as sources of omega-3 fats for heart health and to prevent or treat certain kinds of cancer. Of these plant oils, flaxseed oil is the richest natural source of ALA.

Flaxseed oil in turn has been marketed and sold to the general public for years as a quality source of omega-3 fats. Unfortunately, several studies show that our bodies don't do a very good job of converting the ALA found in flax to EPA and DHA. Men in particular only convert less than 4% of ALA into EPA and less than 0.1% to DHA, making it a very poor source of the more active omega-3 fatty acids for them.

The situation for women is a little more positive. In women, estrogen increases the metabolic machinery needed for converting ALA into EPA and DHA; as a result, young women (in whom estrogen levels are the highest) convert 21% of ALA into EPA and 5-9% into DHA. Postmenopausal women, who have low estrogen levels, are in the same boat as men and make little EPA and almost no DHA.

For optimal health in both men and women it is critical to maintain an appropriate balance of omega-3 and omega-6 fats, but this is especially true for men with prostate cancer. (This dietary imbalance is more extreme than in any other period in human history, and there's a broad consensus among researchers that omega-6 excess coupled with omega-3 deficiencies represents a major health threat.)

The evidence linking EPA and DHA to protection for some of these diseases is strong enough that a recommended daily intake has now been defined. The current recommendation emerged as a consensus from the June 2008 meeting of the Technical Committee on Dietary Lipids of the International Life Sciences Institute North America. These recommendations were based on evidence that these two fatty acids played an important role in preventing fatal cardiovascular disease. The recommendation is that all adults receive at least 250-500 mg per day of EPA plus DHA. Furthermore, it was agreed that humans were not able to satisfy this requirement by ingesting ALA. As flax omega-3 fat is entirely ALA, it is now established that humans cannot satisfy their omega-3 fatty acid needs from this source. The only available sources are fish consumption, fish oil capsules, or DHA extracted from commercially grown algae and marketed by Martek.

Brain and nervous tissue abnormalities figure prominently in the diseases linked to omega-3 fatty acid deficiency and omega-6 fatty acid excess. The retina, which is really an extension of the brain, also requires DHA to function. Our brains actually contain very large amounts of DHA. During human fetal development, large amounts of DHA are required for brain and eye maturation. There are a number of adaptations that help the human infant accumulate the DHA it needs. First, as we discussed before, the surging estrogen levels during pregnancy simulate the conversion of dietary ALA to DHA. Second, the human placenta selectively transports DHA to the fetus. Nevertheless, repeated studies show that in America, fetal and infant development is impaired by the omega-3 fatty acid deficiency so widespread in this country. One study in particular gives us pause. In this study, DHA content of mothers' milk was measured in a range of countries. Japanese women's breast milk had the highest content, consistent with the high fish intake of the Japanese. The lowest levels were seen in Canadian and American mothers. As a result of these studies, supplementation of mothers and infants with DHA is now common.

In adult life, however, fewer factors support adequate brain DHA. As we have just said, fish and fish oil are the only two common sources for DHA, and many Americans do not consume enough fish. This is a real problem for men in particular: The DHA in the brain breaks down and must therefore be replaced. However, men do a very poor job of making DHA from ALA that is widely present in flax, canola, walnuts, and pecans. What this means is that as men age, if they're not getting enough DHA in their diets they may gradually develop DHA deficiency. Diets poor in DHA and other omega-3 fats are associated with a more rapid decline in intellectual function associated with age, increased risk of Alzheimer's, and other forms of dementia.

The recommended daily intake of 250-500 mg of EPA + DHA is based on studies of fatal cardiovascular disease prevention. We do not know enough to establish a daily requirement for optimum neurologic function, but it is most likely to be quite a bit higher than this.

The previous discussion tells us why flaxseed oil is a poor source of omega-3s, but there's actually something a lot more serious and a little more complicated at stake for men and for prostate cancer patients in particular.

In fact, evidence suggests ALA (not just from flaxseed oil, but also from egg yolks and canola oil) may well increase the growth and spread of your cancer. Now, flaxseed may have a slightly different story, since the seeds contain elements other than ALA such as lignans or phytoestrogens.

Our first evidence for flaxseed oil's dangerous effect on prostate cancer comes from a Harvard School of Public Health study that investigated the link between diet and various aspects of health. This study involved monitoring just over 40,000 men followed for over 10 years. This study has led to a number of important publications on prostate cancer, including valuable information on the positive impact of lycopene, vitamin D, and sugar in prostate cancer. Their results on omega-3 fats show that a diet rich in the major plant omega-3 fatty acid, ALA, significantly increased a person's risk of developing advanced prostate cancer. In contrast, omega-3 fats from fish reduced the risk of advanced prostate cancer. Given the sheer size of this patient group, investigators were able to look at a range of interesting issues. One provocative finding was that fish consumption was more beneficial than fish oil supplements, perhaps because fish contain something other than omega-3 fats.

In addition to this large study, there are a number of other studies that have looked at ALA and prostate cancer. The vast majority has either shown an increased risk or at least no benefit from ALA. The bottom line is that it is very hard for us to understand how a health practitioner can continue to advocate plant oils such as flax or canola as viable sources of omega-3 fats. First, as we mentioned earlier, these oils aren't nearly as effective as fish and fish oil at providing any of the heath benefits attributed to omega-3 fatty acids. This is especially true for men. And second, the published medical literature strongly suggests that these plant omega-3 fats increase the risk of developing advanced prostate cancer.

CHAPTER 7
Grilling Meat

There are multiple articles linking red meat to prostate cancer as well as many other cancers. However, the actual risk appears to differ markedly from study to study. Long-term readers of our newsletter, *Prostate Forum*, know that the arachidonic acid content of meat is one factor that led to such a high cancer risk. Arachidonic acid is an omega-6 fatty acid, that promotes the growth and spread of a number of cancers, including prostate cancer. Researchers have demonstrated this by using drugs that block arachidonic acid, such as aspirin, Celebrex, and other NSAIDS to lower the risk of developing clinically significant prostate cancer. Furthermore, Celebrex has been reported to slow the progression of established prostate cancer in these models as well as in patients.

Traditionally, red meat has had a balance between omega-3 and omega-6 fatty acids that were likely to lessen arachidonic acid activation. However, with the modern practice of feeding cattle ruminants like cattle grain (especially corn) the omega-6 content of red meat has increased dramatically and lead to more cancer problems.

It now appears that arachidonic acid content is not the only issue. The way we cook meat also makes a difference. Since 1988, we have known that cooking meat at high temperatures leads to the formation of chemicals that can damage DNA, leading to the development of cancer. This process has been linked to the risk of cancers of the colon, breast, stomach, pancreas and, particularly, the prostate. A study by Tang et al., has brought this into focus. One of the more dangerous chemicals found in cooked meat goes by the abbreviation PhIP, which stands for 2-Amino-1-methyl-6-phenylimida-zo[4,5-b] pyridine. This chemical reacts with DNA, altering its function in a way that favors cancer development. Tang et al., looked for the presence of PhIP bound to the DNA of prostate tissue and prostate cancers in men undergoing radical prostatectomy. They then correlated these results with the patient's preference for consumption of grilled meats. They also looked at how well done the men preferred their meat. There was a very strong statistical correlation between the consumption of grilled red meat and PhIP bound to DNA from the prostate cancer. (For those of you educated in statistics, the p value was 0.002.) In contrast, there was no significant association with the consumption of grilled white meat, which is known to form much less PhIP during cooking. Among the cuts of meat studied, grilled hamburger consumption had the greatest association with DNA damage in the cancer cells. Less PhIP damage was seen in the surrounding non-cancerous prostate cells. Trust us, if you have prostate cancer, the last thing you want is to do anything to fuel further genetic change in your cancer cells. It is the accumulation of genetic damage that causes prostate cancer to become more aggressive and harder to control over time.

Why should the cancer cells be more susceptible to PhIP than the surrounding non-cancerous prostate cells? We think that the best answer comes from William Nelson from Johns Hopkins. He has shown that one of the very first changes that appear in prostate cells after they become cancerous is the loss of glutathione S-transferase P1. This protein protects against PhIP damage and its loss would make the cancer cells much more sensitive to PhIP DNA damage.

In past issues of *Prostate Forum*, we pointed out that the death rate from prostate cancer increased dramatically after World War II. This coincides with the rapid development of fast food restaurants producing grilled hamburger, as well as the growing popularity of charcoal grilling meat at home. Perhaps these trends are linked by the role of PhIP in the development of prostate cancer.

Here is a summary of the evidence that supports a role for PhIP in the development of prostate cancer.

1. PhIP binds to DNA, yielding an easily identified form of damage.

2. Adding PhIP to prostate cancer cells in tissue culture causes this characteristic form of DNA damage.

3. Lack of glutathione S-transferase P1, a defect that appears early in prostate cancer development, makes cells more susceptible to PhIP-induced DNA damage.

4. Human prostate cancer removed by surgery shows PhIP-induced DNA damage directly in proportion to eating red meat cooked at high temperatures.

5. The intake of PhIP is also correlated with the risk of developing prostate cancer.

6. In rodents, PhIP-induced prostate cancer is preceded by inflammation in a manner similar to that seen in humans, where proliferating inflammatory atrophy has been identified as a precursor of prostate cancer.

We are very impressed by the strength of this evidence; it is about as strong a proof as you are likely to get. As you know, scientists have sequenced the human genome and are now identifying many new genes. One area of active research is on genes that inactivate toxic or cancer-causing chemicals. It may well be that we will find that some people are very good at inactivating PhIP and related chemicals. Perhaps this will lead to a pill that would make grilled meat safe!

While involved in prostate cancer development, these chemicals are also implicated in other cancers, such as breast and colon. We should mention that some of these same chemicals are found in cigarette smoke and tail pipe emissions from diesel engines.

How can you reduce or eliminate this risk? You have several options. Of course, you could become a vegetarian or vegan, but most of our readers, as well as most of my patients, are not interested in that option. For the vegetarian, grains and legumes combine well to yield adequate protein. Think of red beans and rice, soy and rice, succotash, pasta, and beans. The classic minestrone from Italy does not contain meat, but commonly combines legumes, grains, and seasonal vegetables. The Mediterranean heart-healthy diet is something of a compromise. In the classic model from Crete, you eat red meat once every 2-4 weeks. You eat fish and white meats more frequently, 1-2 times a week. White chicken or turkey yield lower levels of carcinogens when cooked at high heat, but the carcinogen levels for fish are even lower.

Finally, not all red meat products are equally dangerous. For example, bacon stands out as particularly risky because it is cured with nitrate, smoked, and then seared or baked until crispy. Indeed, the combination of salted, cured meats cooked at high temperatures seems to be particularly bad in terms of carcinogen formation. Another example would be grilled hamburger, as Tang, et al., have shown. In another example, a medium-cooked roast beef has much less PhIP and other carcinogens than a pan-fried steak. Even the details of cooking your meat can make a big difference. If you flip only once, you are exposing at least one side to very high temperatures for quite a while. Flipping the meat multiple times and not letting the meat char or brown excessively will significantly reduce carcinogen formation.

There are also some dietary items that may reduce the formation of, or inactivate, meat carcinogens. They include cruciferous vegetables (cabbage, broccoli, mustard, turnip, kale, and collards); resveratrol; garlic; Asian meat marinades (teriyaki, turmeric, and garlic); soy isoflavones; chlorophyllin; virgin olive oil; and tea polyphenols.

References On Grilled Red Meat

Bogen, K.T., et al., Highly elevated PSA and dietary PhIP intake in a prospective clinic-based study among African Americans. *Prostate Cancer Prostatic Dis*, 2007.

Borowsky, A.D., et al., Inflammation and atrophy precede prostatic neoplasia in a PhIP-induced rat model. *Neoplasia*, 2006. 8(9): p. 708-15.

Coffey, D.S., Similarities of prostate and breast cancer: Evolution, diet, and estrogens. *Urology*, 2001. 57(4 Suppl 1): p. 31-8.

Cross, A.J., et al., A prospective study of meat and meat mutagens and prostate cancer risk. *Cancer Res*, 2005. 65(24): p. 11779-84.

Dingley, K.H., et al., Effect of dietary constituents with chemopreventive potential on adduct formation of a low dose of the heterocyclic amines PhIP and IQ and phase II hepatic enzymes. *Nutr Cancer*, 2003. 46(2): p. 212-21.

El-Zein, R., et al., Human sensitivity to PhIP: a novel marker for prostate cancer risk. *Mutat Res*, 2006. 601(1-2): p. 1-10.

Hikosaka, A., et al., Inhibitory effects of soy isoflavones on rat prostate carcinogenesis induced by 2-amino-1-methyl-6-phenylimidazo[4,5-b]pyridine(PhIP). *Carcinogenesis*, 2004. 25(3): p. 381-7.

Nakai, Y., W.G. Nelson, and A.M. De Marzo, The dietary charred meat carcinogen 2-amino-1-methyl-6- phenylimidazo[4,5-b]pyridine acts as both a tumor initiator and promoter in the rat ventral prostate. *Cancer Res*, 2007. 67(3): p. 1378-84.

Nelson, C.P., et al., Protection against 2-hydrox- yamino-1-methyl-6-phenylimidazo[4,5-b]pyridine cytotoxici-ty and DNA adduct formation in human prostate by glutathione S-transferase P1. *Cancer Res*, 2001. 61(1): p. 103-9.

Tang, D., et al., Grilled Meat Consumption and PhIP- DNA Adducts in Prostate Carcinogenesis. *Cancer Epidemiol Biomarkers Prev*, 2007. 16(4): p. 803-8.

Tappel, A., Heme of consumed red meat can act as a catalyst of oxidative damage and could initiate colon, breast and prostate cancers, heart disease and other diseases. *Med Hypotheses*, 2007. 68(3): p. 562-4.

Williams, J.A., et al., Metabolic activation of carcinogens and expression of various cytochromes P450 in human prostate tissue. *Carcinogenesis*, 2000. 21(9): p. 1683-9.

Wilson, C., et al., Diallyl sulfide inhibits PhIP-induced DNA strand breaks in normal human breast epithelial cells. *Oncol Rep*, 2007. 17(4): p. 807-11.

CHAPTER 8

Scientific Support for the Mediterranean Diet

The New Prostate Cancer Nutrition Book presents a cuisine based on the Mediterranean diet. At various points in the book, we mention that this diet has been studied extensively in clinical trials. This fact played an important role in our decision to focus on the Mediterranean diet. In this section, we will cover some of the key clinical trials that influenced our thinking on diet. We'll go into a detailed definition of the version of the Mediterranean diet we recommend in later chapters, but for now we're going to discuss the scientific evidence behind it.

The first randomized controlled trial worth mentioning is the Lyon Diet Heart trial, published in 1999. In this trial, 605 people who had just had their first heart attack were randomized into two groups: 1) a prudent Western diet similar to the American Heart Association Step 1 diet versus 2) a diet patterned after that on the island of Crete. Crete was chosen because it is a well-studied version of the Mediterranean diet and associated with longevity and a low-risk of cardiovascular disease. The results were reported after a mean follow-up of 46 months. There were 44 cases of cardiac death or recurrent heart attack in the control arm and 14 in the Mediterranean diet arm. If you include incidents of unstable angina, stroke, heart failure, and embolism, there were 90 cases in the control arm and 27 in the Mediterranean diet arm. Obviously, this is a very impressive benefit. Of note, there was also a 60% reduction in the incidence of cancer in the Mediterranean diet arm.

One aspect of this trial warrants additional comment. To increase the omega-3 fatty acid content of the diet, canola oil was added to contribute 1,000 mg of alpha linolenic acid. As discussed elsewhere, we now know that alpha linolenic acid is markedly less effective than the omega-3 fats from fish, DHA, and EPA. If you're interested in looking at the study yourself, the citation is D Lorgeril, et al., "Mediterranean diet, traditional risk factors, and the rate of cardiovascular complications after myocardial infarction: final report of the Lyon Diet Heart Study" *Circulation* 99: 779-785, 1999.

The second study of interest was the GISSI-Prevenzione trial. This was not a randomized controlled trial, but nevertheless the results have proved useful. This trial was conducted at 172 centers in the Italian public health system and involved 11,323 people with a history of a heart attack. The subjects were advised to increase their consumption of fish, fruit, vegetables, and olive oil. They were also advised to take 1,000 mg of fish oil a day. Actual diet composition was assessed at baseline, 6, 18, and 42 months. The patients were also treated with state of the art cardiac drugs, including statins. Increases in each of the major food items listed were associated with a reduced risk of cardiovascular issues, cardiac death, sudden death, and overall death rates. The major finding was that adding 1,000 mg of fish oil resulted in an additional 20% drop in overall deaths and a 45% reduction in the risk of sudden death. This contribution of fish oil was impressive because it appeared over and above the benefit of the Mediterranean diet and a state of the art drug program, including statins.

The best commentary we can find on this clinical study was an editorial by Alexander Leaf published in *Circulation*. The full text of this editorial is available online and is one of the best short reviews of the need to reduce omega-6 and increase omega-3 content of your diet.

In case you're interested, the citations for the three studies are: R. Marchioli, et al. "Mediterranean diet and all-causes mortality after myocardial infarction: results from the GISSI-Prevenzione trial" *European Journal Clinical Nutrition* 57: 604-611, 2003; R. Marchioli, et al. "Early Protection Against Sudden Death by n-3 Polyunsaturated Fatty Acids After Myocardial

Infarction" *Circulation* 105: 1897-1903, 2002; and Alexander Leaf "On the Reanalysis of the GISSI-Prevenzione" *Circulation* 105: 1874-1875, 2002.

The next trial is of interest for two reasons. First, it is a large randomized controlled trial. Second, it took place outside the Mediterranean basin: India to be specific. The control diet was a local diet equivalent to the prudent Step 1 diet used in the Lyon study. The experimental diet was designed to duplicate the concepts behind the Mediterranean diet using foods available in India that were rich in whole grains, fruits, vegetables and nuts. Mustard or soybean oil was used rather than olive oil. The experimental diet had twice the omega-3 content as the control arm, largely as alpha linolenic acid. One thousand subjects with angina, heart attack, or significant risk factors for cardiovascular disease were randomized. There were 76 cardiac events in the control arm compared with 39 in the Indo-Mediterranean arm. The number of sudden deaths was also reduced from 16 to 6.

Here's the citation: Singh, R.B et al. "Effect of an Indo-Mediterranean diet on progression of coronary artery disease in high-risk patients: a randomized single-blind trial" *The Lancet* 360: 1455-1461, 2002.

In the interest of further geographical diversity, the next clinical trial, PREDIMED, was conducted in Spain. This study involved 1,551 people with diabetes or 3 or more cardiovascular risk factors. In addition to the control low fat diet arm, there were two Mediterranean diet arms–one with a liter a week of olive oil and the other 30 grams of nuts a day. This trial is still early and only intermediate endpoints have been described. However, the early results are very interesting in that they suggest that the risk of diabetes and metabolic syndrome may be reduced. After a median follow-up of 4 years, the risk of diabetes was reduced by 52% by the Mediterranean diet. As of yet, there is no significant difference between nuts and olive oil. Here's the citation: Salas-Salvado, J, et al. "Reduction in the incidence of type 3 diabetes with the Mediterranean diet: results of the PREDIMED-Reus nutrition intervention randomized trial" *Diabetes Care* 34: 14-19, 2010.

There are many other trials that could be discussed, but we think citing a few comprehensive review papers can cover these. First, the review by Esposito, K, et al. "Prevention and control of type 2 diabetes by Mediterranean diet: a systematic review" *Diabetes Research Clinical Practice* 89: 97-102, 2010 found that the literature consistently documents that the Mediterranean diet helps prevent type 2 diabetes, improves glycemic control, and reduces cardiovascular risk.

This review also merits discussion: Esposito, K, et al. "Mediterranean diet and weight loss: meta-analysis of randomized controlled trials" *Metabolic Syndrome Related Disorders* 9: 1-12, 2010. The Mediterranean diet is 30-40% fat by calories, leading to concern about weight gain. This review covered studies reporting the impact of the Mediterranean diet on weight loss. They found this diet supported weight loss if patients remained on it for greater than 6 months. Weight loss was further enhanced if the diet was combined with calorie restriction and/or exercise, which is hardly surprising.

Metabolic syndrome is the combination of excessive abdominal fat, elevated blood sugar and hypertension that is increasingly common in the United States. Metabolic syndrome is associated with a dramatic increased risk of diabetes, heart disease, stroke and death. This review found convincing evidence of benefit for the Mediterranean diet in multiple clinical trials. This is the citation: Kastorini, C.M. et al. "The effect of Mediterranean diet on metabolic syndrome and its components: a meta-analysis of 50 studies and 534,906 individuals" *Journal American College of Cardiology* 57: 1299-1313, 2011.

CHAPTER 9

Exercise

In this chapter we'll teach you how to use exercise to trigger your body's innate repair programs needed to promote optimal health. Humans come from a long line of endurance predators who had to cover great distances to get a meal. As you might expect, our biology is fine-tuned to support this activity. With each bout of exercise, repair programs are triggered that not only fix any damage caused during the exercise, but also lessen degeneration that aging might cause. This repair involves muscles, but also tendons, blood vessels, heart, and brain. Nature has its own way of telling us this. People consistently report a feeling of well-being after they exercise. They may be tired or depressed when they start, but after a period of time these problems tend to fade away. This is nature's way of saying, "job well done."

Our thinking on exercise has been heavily influenced by the HOPE trial. The HOPE study involved 2,300 men and women between the ages of 70-90. The investigators looked at the relationship between four lifestyle choices and survival: smoking, moderate alcohol consumption, Mediterranean diet, and exercise. They found that people who exercised for at least 30 minutes a day had a 25-30% drop in overall death rate. Randomized controlled trials have also shown that exercise reduces the risk of cancer death rate, obesity, diabetes, hypertension, and heart attack. Besides, exercise reduces the risk of cancer of the colon and other malignancies, such as breast cancer. While it does not appear to reduce the risk of prostate cancer, it can have a profound impact on the quality of life and outcome of treatment for men with prostate cancer.

Men on hormonal therapy and people on chemotherapy and radiation tend to lose muscle strength and muscle mass.

People with severe heart disease or emphysema also lose muscle mass and this further impairs their function. Exercise helps many people control hypertension and diabetes. If you adopt a program of aerobic exercise and resistance exercise, you can limit your loss of muscle strength and muscle mass. Your recovery from treatment will likewise be more rapid.

Because we follow patients for many years at American Institute For Diseases of the Prostate (www.prostateteam. com), we have the privilege of watching them age. Time and again, I am struck by how those who do not exercise regularly become progressively impaired as they age. Most patients I see at age 70 are fully able to conduct their lives whether they have exercised or not. In contrast, by the time they reach age 80, with rare exceptions, only those patients who exercise and watch their diet are fully functional. First, those who do not exercise lose balance to the point where they are constantly at risk for falling. Second, the strength of their hip muscles have weakened to the point where it is difficult to get out of chairs or climb stairs. Often, the shoulder rotator cuff muscles have weakened to the point where they no longer protect the joint from damage and must be surgically repaired with a long period of physical therapy treatment.

All of us here at *Prostate Forum* personally fear dementia much more than physical decline. My own bout with aggressive cancer treatments left me disabled for more than a year. I found that I could enjoy life while reading books and enjoying the company of friends and family. Dementia steals all of that from you. In fact, we now know that the brain is very dynamic and responds to being used as much as any muscle. We also know that exercise plays a major role in helping your brain renew itself. Those who exercise have better memories, are better coordinated, and are better able to solve problems that arise.

Studies show that active people have higher basal metabolisms than sedentary people. Standing, walking, bending, and twisting all contribute to burning calories. At a very basic level, get out of your chair. If you must sit, fidget around in your seat and move your hands and legs. If you work at a computer all day, try standing or sitting on a large exercise ball.

Aerobic exercise can be as simple or as elaborate as you want to make it. At a minimum, you should aim for at least 30 minutes of brisk walking outside, in a health club, or in a large indoor mall. In my own case, Rose and I bought a treadmill and placed it in front of a television set. Now, even when I finish work at 9 pm, I can still get my time in.

Establishing An Exercise Program

As a key first step, make sure your exercise program has the proper balance between aerobic exercise to maintain cardiovascular health and resistance exercise to make sure the muscles important to every day life maintain their function.

Aerobic exercise

Start out gently; it is better to underestimate what you can do at first. Often people begin so aggressively that they cannot continue the exercise routine they have set out to accomplish. You can get tremendous benefit from a very simple, basic program. It is now clear that just 30 minutes of brisk walking can do wonders for your long-term health. From the HOPE trial, we know that even 30 minutes of gardening will do the job. Some of you have trouble walking because of joint problems. Most exercise facilities have recumbent bicycles and these offer a chance to exercise with no stress on your back at all. Recumbent bicycles also offer you a chance to start off at a very slow pace with even less energy output than walking. Most health clubs also offer programs in aquatic exercise and these are a wonderful option if you are overweight or have joint problems.

Exercise can become addictive; it triggers some of the same parts of the brain that heroin does. One goal of a program is to get you addicted to exercise so that you will look forward to your daily fix. If you are already addicted to drugs, alcohol, or tobacco, exercise can become a healthy substitute. For this to happen, you need to avoid the traps that block people from continuing their exercise program long enough for you to let the addiction take hold.

Obstacles To Exercising

If you exercise outdoors, you will soon face the problem of bad weather. There are only a few places in the United States where every day is pleasant outside. Here in Charlottesville, Virginia where our central offices are located, we have ice and snow in January and February and 90 degree days June through August. Also, the winter days are short enough that if you work, you will be exercising outdoors in the dark. When you find it unpleasant to go outside, you need to find a convenient place to work out indoors.

For most people, health clubs represent the best answer. They are set up to make exercise fun. There are classes you can join that can be great fun and teach you new skills. You might even hire a personal trainer to ensure that your program is well thought out and balanced. Furthermore, people often do more at the start of an exercise routine when they are part of a group. Clubs will have a wide range of machines that you can use for aerobic exercise so you can pick something that fits your needs. Recumbent bicycles are commonly available. Elliptical machines duplicate many of the motions involved in running, but without the impact. Treadmills are available and while people use these for running, we suggest you initially focus on walking. When I started exercising again after radiation and hormonal therapy, walking on a treadmill formed the basis of my program. In addition to adjusting the pace, you can intensify your program by increasing the slope of the treadmill. Stair climbing machines are also widely available and these can give you exercise intensity that ranges from mild to Olympic trial intensity without the impact of running. Stair climbing machines excel at strengthening the very muscles of the hip needed to get out of a chair or climb stairs. This makes them the perfect antidote to the losses of aging. These health clubs commonly have television sets in front of the machine, and if you bring headphones, listening to a show or music can help with the boredom of being inside and on a machine. Additionally, health clubs have resistance exercise machines and free weights. Free weights are a great option for resistance training. You can transfer these exercises to home with the purchase of a few weights.

If you do not have access to a health club, we can think of two options. Shopping malls make a nice place to walk in bad weather. In fact, in many parts of the country, large malls have walking clubs of seniors who get together several times a week to walk. While walking the mall, you will have a chance to make new friends and have a good time; at the end of the session, mall walkers will commonly have lunch together.

Finding time is the other primary obstacle to developing and maintaining a good exercise program. As we mentioned earlier, during the workweek, I often finish patient consultations as late as 9 pm; it is always dark outside and the health clubs in Central Virginia are closed by then as well. Over the years, Rose and I have gradually built quite an exercise room in their home by purchasing used equipment we found advertised in local papers. This way I can exercise no matter when I finish work in the evenings. If you do not have the space to set up a room like this, a few weights and a yoga mat are all you'll need to get your resistance exercise. An exercise video—there are hundreds to choose from—can substitute for the cardio portion of your program on days you can't make it either outside for a walk or to the health club.

Fine-Tuning Your Exercise Program

You can stay with the 30 minutes of mild aerobic exercise and gain important benefits from walking, running, biking, hiking, or swimming; however, the benefits of exercise increase with duration. Sixty minutes of aerobic exercise is better than thirty minutes of exercise, especially for weight control. In turn, ninety minutes is more beneficial than sixty minutes. In practice, few are likely to put this time in on a daily basis; yet, enormous benefit can be achieved by going long once or twice a week. In competitive endurance sports, it is recognized that going long at least once a week not only improves endurance, but also causes a steady increase in the intensity you can sustain in your daily exercise.

In the history of endurance sports, one approach to excellence was just to run longer and longer without regard to intensity. This approach has limited returns and is not very practical unless you are willing to spend all of your time exercising. Even ninety minutes involves more time than most are willing to spend. What is the path out of this dilemma? The answer is what is called interval training. This involves periodic bouts of intense exercise thrown into the middle of a typical daily training session.

The development of interval training is an interesting one in the history of sports. The movement came to a peak in the early 1950s. The first major episode was the 1952 Olympics, when Emil Zatopek won the 5,000 meters, 10,000 meters and the marathon gold medals. He also broke the Olympic record in each of those events. No one since has duplicated that triple win let alone record time. His training involved nothing but running 400 meters at a rapid pace followed by a recovery lap and then another fast lap.

The second major event that helped establish interval training as a method to increase endurance occurred 2 years later in 1954, when Roger Bannister became the first man to break four minutes for a mile. What was shocking at the time and is today was that he did this on very light training compared to other runners of his time. His success was based on intensive interval training. I was just starting out on the high school track team at the time and remember well the impact Zatopec and Bannister had on how people thought about training.

Following these successes, interval training has come to dominate every endurance sport including running, swimming, and bicycle racing. For us, however, it is more important to note that interval training has now been shown to be the best approach to cardiac rehabilitation and improving the function of patients with emphysema.

Before we get into the details of how you can use interval training, there are several things you need to address before you start.

Heart Rate Monitors

You can safely exercise by just limiting yourself to a pace that is comfortable. However, there are many advantages to controlling your pace with a heart rate monitor as most of the scientific literature on exercise discusses pace as a percent of maximal heart rate. Excellent heart rate monitors are available for under $100. These include two parts: one is a strap that goes around your chest and records your heartbeat; the other is a monitor on your wrist that displays your current heart rate. Many exercise machines are able to read the transmission of your chest strap and show your heart rate during exercise. Some will adjust the speed of the treadmill to keep your heart rate at a target level.

Many heart rate monitors come with target heart rates based on age. The tables that specify heart rates based upon age have no scientific basis and are potentially dangerous. It is much better to have your maximal heart rate measured and then to exercise at a percent of your maximal heart rate. This means a visit to a cardiologist for a stress test as part of the process of getting your maximal heart rate measured. This is a very good idea, as you really should have a stress test done before increasing your exercise intensity.

With the maximal heart rate measured, you will want to do most of your exercise above 60% of maximal heart rate. Real development of aerobic capacity starts at 70-75% of maximal heart rate. A good place to start with intervals would be 1 minute at 80% of your maximal heart rate with five minutes of slower paced (70%) exercise between each intense episode. You can then work up to five minutes of intensity with five minutes of recovery. If you find you like this and would like to explore heart rate based training further, I recommend you get *The Heart Rate Guidebook to Heart Zones Training* by Sally Edwards. I have found this to be the most useful introduction to this form of training.

For most of you reading this book, one long workout on the weekend and one or two interval sessions during the week is a good way to improve cardiovascular fitness.

Starting Interval Training

We're going to assume you have had your stress test and have a heart rate monitor. If you are new to exercise, it is important that you have at least 6 months of pure endurance training under your belt before you start this. Also, it is very important to be patient and progress gradually. When you increase intensity by a step, it takes your body a full six weeks to respond to that increase in intensity. Therefore, we plan for you to spend at least 6 weeks at each step and you would certainly do fine with 8 weeks at each step. Time and again, we have seen people hurt themselves, get discouraged, and stop completely because they pushed too hard too fast.

Here's a sample interval-training schedule:

Day	Time
Monday	30 min
Tuesday	60 min
Wednesday	30 min
Thursday	60 min
Friday	30 min
Saturday	90 min
Sunday	Rest

In the days without intervals, your time is spent at 70% of maximal heart rate. On the days of intervals, you will warm up for 20 minutes at 70% of maximum heart rate.

For Step 1, at 20 minutes, go at 80% of maximal heart rate for one minute and then slow back down to 70% until you hit the 30-minute mark. At this point, you do another 1 minute at 80% and then drop back down to 70%. This process is continued in 10-minute blocks until you hit 60 minutes.

Every 6 to 8 weeks, you increase the time at speed by one minute until you spend 5 minutes at 80% and 5 minutes at 70% for each ten-minute block.

Resistance Exercises and Stretching

Resistance exercises are easily described as putting a muscle under stress with external weights, elastic bands, and body weight. Why do resistance exercises? Basically, two reasons come to mind: resistance exercises decrease bone loss, and in many cases increase bone density, and they increase muscle tone and strength. Bone density is an important index as we age because bone loss often results in osteopenia and osteoporosis. Therefore, the bones affected will fracture under undo stress, and if the osteoporosis is severe, can easily break. Muscular strength and tone are important for everyday life as we lift, carry, bend, climb stairs, walk, and sit in and get out of chairs. The stronger our muscles are the easier daily tasks are to complete. It is especially important to keep the arm, shoulder, hips, back, and leg muscles strong. Muscle tone comes with strengthening muscles. Because these exercises involve the large muscle groups of the trunk, hips, and thighs, they play a critical role in building aerobic fitness as well as providing muscle mass to burn calories. Resistance exercises should be done at least three times a week.

You should begin a resistance exercise program with low weight poundage and eventually build the amount of weight. Many muscle groups can be strengthened with free weights or hand weights. For example, the arm and shoulder muscles can be strengthened with a simple hand weight for biceps, triceps, deltoids, rhomboids, trapezius, and other scapular muscles. Your body, as resistance or weight, is employed when you do lunges and squats, pull-ups, push-ups, and curls for hip, upper and lower legs, abdominal and shoulder and back muscles.

Stretching is important in combating the effects of everyday life. We sometimes spend part of our days sitting at our computers, sitting for long periods of time commuting, or standing for long periods of time. A routine of stretching for all muscle groups is a good habit to form. Make sure to stretch your back, hip, shoulder, and leg muscles. These stretching routines should be a part of the overall program developed for you.

Of course, the best way to go about developing a resistance exercise and stretching program is to join a health club and have a personal trainer set up a program that incorporates the proper form and techniques. Find a routine that suits your needs.

Weight Loss

Our goal is to guide you toward a healthy diet. It is our conviction that it is very important that you first establish a healthy diet and exercise program. You should only start to focus on losing weight after these other elements are in place. If you proceed in this fashion, switching to a weight loss program is relatively easy.

We're sure you are all aware of the epidemic of obesity taking place in the United States today. I have watched this epidemic take hold during my career in medicine and have spent much time reflecting on the causes. I think the major forces at work are obvious. First, the portion size of meals at restaurants and, probably at home, have increased dramatically. Second, it is easier and easier to be physically inactive. Television, the Internet, and the car have combined to allow us to do our business and pleasure by the seat of our pants. However, I also think that there have been some important changes in the American diet that have helped set up the obesity epidemic.

It is now very clear that the "low fat" diets that have been advocated seriously damage the health of many men and women. When people set out to restrict fats of all kinds, they will typically increase the amount of carbohydrates they eat. Many of us are poorly equipped genetically to handle this high carbohydrate load. The result is the development of insulin resistance, belly fat, hypertension, elevated serum triglycerides, and an increase in fasting blood sugar. Taken to an extreme, this can lead to the development of metabolic syndrome, diabetes, heart attack, stroke, and liver failure.

There is an added problem with carbohydrates. Sugar is addictive. When alcoholics stop drinking, they often gain weight because of a dramatic increase in the intake of sweets. Sweet-tasting foods trigger some of the same circuits that used to be triggered by alcohol. Even people who are not alcoholics will often crave sweets and act as if they are addicted to them. The modern fast food restaurant offers the sweets addict a rapid fix. For very little money, you can get a full quart of soda loaded with sugar, a pastry or two and ice cream for dessert. I still remember a patient who had gained 52 pounds in the 52 weeks since his last visit. When I asked what the man had had for breakfast, he mentioned a quart of full sugar soda and twelve glazed donuts! Not a practical longevity plan to say the least.

So, before you actually start trying to lose weight, you need to bring your carbohydrate intake into balance.

Among the popular diets the two that come closest to providing useful guidance are the *Zone Diet* and the *South Beach* diet. We prefer the *Zone Diet* approach because it is much easier to implement and emphasizes a generally healthy diet. If you want to go into the *Zone Diet* in greater detail, Berry Sears has quite a few books on sale at Amazon.com. This quote from Berry Sears is a nice introduction to the simplicity of his diet concept.

"Eat as much protein as the palm of your hand, as much non-starchy raw vegetables as you can stand for the vitamins, enough carbohydrates to maintain mental clarity because the brain runs on glucose, and enough monounsaturated oils to keep feelings of hunger away."

The heart of his program is that each meal should have a balance between protein, carbohydrate, and heart-healthy fat. A second principle is that you should have frequent meals during the day rather than three large meals. He recommends that in addition to breakfast, you have a small snack mid-afternoon and at bedtime. Furthermore, you can consider a midmorning snack. Each of these snacks must also be balanced between protein, carbohydrate, and fat. The third principle is that the fat should not be animal fat, but rather monounsaturated fat, such as those we recommend in this book. He also stresses the importance of fish and fish oil. In essence, his whole program is easy to fit into our Mediterranean diet recommendations and he supplements these with specific recommendations on the serving portions.

In my experience, most of my patients start to go wrong with breakfast. A typical breakfast of cereal with milk, some fruit, and perhaps toast is nearly all carbohydrate and is lacking in both protein and heart-healthy fat. Instead, most patients would do better with 20-30 grams of protein, 6-10 almonds, and 30-40 grams of carbohydrate. In some men who are already having trouble with blood sugar, they might want to reduce the carbohydrate intake further. For example, when I started my own weight loss program after gaining weight when I was on hormonal therapy, my breakfast was 1/2 to 3/4 cup of Eggbeaters, 6-8 almonds, and an apple.

Soy powder is readily available and can also offer 20 or 25 grams of healthy protein per scoop. It can easily be combined with frozen fruit (red-purple berries would be great) to give you a smoothie with the proper amounts of protein and carbohydrate. You can either throw in the nuts (almonds, cashews, hazelnuts, pistachios) or eat the nuts separately. Lunch and dinner are much easier and Dr. Sears' quote is a very nice summary of how to approach each meal.

Exercise is an important adjunct to this diet change. However, many of my patients think exercise can counter dietary excesses. This is not true. Exercise without diet does very little in terms of weight loss. You can continue to progress down the road to diabetes, heart attack and stroke if you do not change your diet. As one patient told me years ago, he found he could out eat any exercise program! This did not surprise me, as it is true for nearly everyone. Get your diet in control first and foremost, and then gradually add exercise.

Weight Loss Rules of Thumb
Each meal: 20-25 grams of protein, 1 tablespoon of nuts,
    25-30 grams of carbohydrate.
Snacks: 1/2 an apple, 3 nuts, 7 grams of protein.

After you are on this diet for a while, you may find your need for carbohydrates is lower or higher than this average. People with a strong family history of diabetes and/or visceral obesity may find they do better with less carbohydrate and more nuts. People engaged in intense exercise programs may need more carbohydrates.

First, get into the habit of healthy eating. If you need to lose weight, after a few months, you can start to reduce the amount of calories in each meal. There are two practices which can help you lose weight: reduce the serving size of each meal you eat; and increase the volume of non-starchy vegetables to keep your stomach full.

CHAPTER 10

What You Should Eat

Do you have to change your whole diet? That, of course, depends on what you eat now. If you exist on steak, fries, ice cream, and donuts with only a sprinkling of vegetables, then yes, you do have to change your entire diet. If you eat chicken, fish, vegetables, and fruits, you probably only need to adjust some items. The goal is to achieve balance between fats, carbohydrates, and proteins. Eat healthy foods cooked in healthy ways.

Inconsistencies abound in the diet world with conflicting information; some of these inconsistencies are based in fact, but most are based on fiction or opinion. We have moderated our stance on diet as new information became available on cardiovascular disease, diabetes, and cancer. For example, we no longer believe that a very low fat diet is best for our health. What we know now can impact the quality and length of your life. Again: balance protein, carbohydrates, and fat. Eliminating one of these food groups leads to poor health because all three are essential for the body to maintain optimal function. We know that the type of fats we eat affects cardiovascular health, diabetes, and cancer. Eating foods high in omega-6 fatty acids eventually leads to poor health. Therefore, knowing the fat composition of foods becomes an essential part of becoming and staying healthy.

No matter what type of diet you elect to use, make sure it is based on the best available evidence and that your diet is accompanied by a good exercise and relaxation routine. The good habits you establish and maintain early in life will pay enormous dividends as you age. The benefits of dietary changes can be experienced later in life and can sometimes reverse the effects of an earlier rocky start. But the earlier you adopt a healthy lifestyle the fewer health problems you will experience down the road.

Here are several easy dietary changes you can make immediately.

Red Meat

You can change your diet significantly by eliminating red meat and grilled meats. After being raised in a pasture, cattle are usually finished in a feedlot and consume feed that contains fat detrimental to heart-health and that may fuel the growth and incidence of various cancers. These fats harm your blood vessels and cause numerous diseases to develop.

Why does beef fat negatively impact your health? Cattle are usually finished on grains containing omega-6 fatty acids, such as corn. To make matters worse, many people cook beef by grilling or browning it, which causes the outside of the meat to burn, producing carcinogenic material that affects the incidence of cancer. We think cattle raised only on grasses may be healthier, but randomized controlled trials have not been conducted and reported. The jury is still out on keeping red meat in your diet; therefore, it is best to eliminate red meat products such as beef, lamb, and pork. If you must have a treat every now and then, which means infrequently, eat grass-fed livestock and do not char the meat.

We are leery of farm-raised fish and crustaceans, with the exception of rainbow trout. Why? Most farm-raised fish are fed grains and develop omega-6 fatty acids as a result. Fish in the oceans, rivers, and lakes eat insects, other marine life, algae, and plant material. They do not eat corn and grains. Cold-water ocean fish develop omega-3 fatty acids and not omega-6 fatty acids. That's why ocean-caught fish are healthier for us than farm-raised fish. Farm-raised trout, on the other hand, are fed other foods and therefore are free from the omega-6 fatty acids.

If the fat content of wild versus farm-raised fish won't sway you, the taste will. Salmon in particular was meant to swim unobstructed from creek to ocean to creek, and you can taste the difference in a wild salmon's tender flaky flesh and flavor depth. You can actually see the salmon's life in its flesh: wild salmon has streaks of fat between the muscle, which gives the fish its characteristic tenderness and flavor; farm-raised salmon has thin weak lines of fat, which make it more likely to dry out in the cooking process. There are a few fish farms that produce a good product; if you don't have time to research a farm's methods, ask your fish monger where the farm is located and what methods they practice. What is the fish fed? Does the feed contain antibiotics or dyes? Is the feed organic? If the fishmonger cannot answer these questions, or provide you with someone to contact who has answers, do not purchase the farmed salmon.

When we raise our animals (cows, sheep, pigs) and fish on corn, grains, and growth hormones to accelerate growth, we cause many problems. In cattle, omega-6 fatty acids and ulcers develop. The fatty acid is a problem unto itself. The ulcers an animal develops from eating grains necessitate antibiotics to combat infection. Corn-fed, and administered antibiotics and growth hormones, the hamburger that ends up on your plate is dangerous for you. Further, much is still unknown about the effects of antibiotics and growth hormones on our health. In the meantime, it is best to simply eliminate red meats and pork from your diet.

As we just noted, farmed fish can result in an unhealthy fatty acid composition. To increase our odds of eating healthy foods we eliminate farm-raised fish, seafood, and red meat products raised on corn and grains, growth hormones, and antibiotics.

Healthy & Unhealthy Oils

Other changes you can incorporate are to eat and use only monounsaturated oils in cooking such as olive, hazelnut, almond, and avocado oils. Other nuts that are rich in monounsaturated fats are pistachio, cashews, and macadamia nuts. Corn oil, and to a lesser extent, sunflower seed oil, cottonseed oil, and soybean oil consist mainly of omega-6 fatty acids, which we know are detrimental to our health. Flaxseed and canola oils are high in an omega-3 fat that is not effective for human nutrition and has been associated with an increased risk for prostate cancer. (Again, for more information on flaxseed oil, read our booklet *Flaxseed: Panacea or Poison*, available at http://www.prostateforum.com/flaxseed.html).

It is very easy to adopt olive oil as your main source of oil. There are light olive oils for sautéing and heavier olive oils for flavoring dishes, vinaigrettes, and for other salad dressings. Today olive oils are available from Australia, California, Sardinia, Greece, France, Sicily, and various regions in Italy. We continue to experiment with new oils as we encounter them. Each region has its own method of pressing, which allows distinct flavors to develop. Experiment to find the olive oils you like best.

Vegetables & Fruits

A refrain every child has heard is "Eat your vegetables!" But why? Low in fat, vegetables and fruits contain many vitamins and minerals, fiber, and antioxidants. They are easy to cook and provide healthy and colorful carbohydrates. Potatoes, yams, carrots, and grains (rice, barley, wheat, oats, millet, and others) provide carbohydrates and fiber. The combination of vegetables and grains can provide an array of vitamins and minerals, and supply us with many complex carbohydrates. Many contain a high concentration of sugars and should be eaten in moderation. Fruits are an essential part of any diet and especially berries and pomegranates contain many powerful antioxidants.

We recommend organically raised fruits, vegetables, and poultry. Why? We are leery of the pesticides, fertilizers, and weed killers used to grow vegetables, fruits, and grains. Most of these chemicals are linked to poor health. If possible, grow your own organically raised produce, and whenever possible, buy organically raised products from the grocery stores and farmers' markets. Some fruits and vegetables are sprayed more often than others. Below is a list of the pesticide load of certain fruits and vegetables, ranked from highest to lowest pesticide content, tested by the Environmental Working Group.

Pesticide Load Of Popular Fruit & Vegetables

Most dangerous. . . . . *Highest pesticide load*
1	Peach	100
2	Apple	93
3	Sweet Bell Pepper	83
4	Celery	82
5	Nectarine	81
6	Strawberries	80
7	Cherries	73
8	Kale	69
9	Lettuce	67
10	Grapes - Imported	66
11	Carrot	63
12	Pear	63
13	Collard Greens	60
14	Spinach	58
15	Potato	56
16	Green Beans	53
17	Summer Squash	53
18	Pepper	51
19	Cucumber	50
20	Raspberries	46
21	Grapes - Domestic	44
22	Plum	44
23	Orange	44
24	Cauliflower	39
25	Tangerine	37
26	Mushrooms	36

27 Banana 34
28 Winter Squash 34
29 Cantaloupe 33
30 Cranberries 33
31 Honeydew Melon 30
32 Grapefruit 29
33 Sweet Potato 29
34 Tomato 29
35 Broccoli 28
36 Watermelon 26
37 Papaya 20
38 Eggplant 20
39 Cabbage 17
40 Kiwi 13
41 Sweet Peas - Frozen 10
42 Asparagus 10
43 Mango. 9
44 Pineapple 7
45 Sweet Corn - Frozen 2
46 Avocado 1
47 Onion 1
Safest. . . . . .Lowest pesticide load

Note: EWG ranked a total of 47 different fruits and vegetables but grapes are listed twice because they looked at both domestic and imported samples.

Vegetarian & Vegan Diets

A great deal has been written about eliminating animal products from your diet. What do we think? Ten years ago, we followed a vegetarian diet and were leaning toward a vegan diet because the evidence showed that these types of diets resulted in fewer cardiovascular problems and cancer. Now we know that wild, cold water fish can be a good addition to our meals and as long as we eliminate omega-6 fatty acids and don't char our meats we can reduce our risk of heart disease and cancer.

But there are many who believe that a vegetarian type diet is the best policy to follow for social and religious reasons. We will explain the principles behind these diets and offer general guidelines.

A lacto-vegetarian consumes grains, cereals, legumes, vegetables, fruits, and dairy products, but no eggs. A lacto-ovo vegetarian eats dairy products and eggs. To keep this type of diet healthy you should use low- or no-fat dairy products. Egg whites can be consumed liberally, because they are the purest form of protein with no fat or cholesterol. Egg yolks contain fats that reflect the diet of the chickens producing the eggs. If the chicken is fed a diet rich in corn, the resulting egg will be high in omega-6 fats. Chicken feed that contains a combination of grains and beans such as oats, wheat, barley, soybeans, peas, millet, or other grains instead of corn will have much less omega-6 fatty acid content. Rose raises chickens and has developed a feed free from corn that contains oats, soybean, millet, fishmeal, and algae. Her chickens are free-range and pastured on fresh fields throughout the year, consuming worms and insects in the Spring, Summer, and Fall. The eggs her chickens produce on this feed are now being tested.

A vegan eats grains, cereals, legumes, vegetables, and fruits but no dairy products or eggs. To be healthy and maintain a diet that includes all the vitamins and minerals your body needs you should learn to combine foods correctly. Have a serving of brown rice with legumes (lentils, garbanzo beans, soybeans, navy beans, etc.). Be creative and try other grains with legumes, sea vegetables, or greens. Eat liberal amounts of cooked tomatoes, beets, and yellow vegetables, in addition to oranges, apricots, and pumpkin as they contain compounds called carotenoids (the pigments in fruits and vegetables that give them their bright color) and are excellent sources of antioxidants. A vegan or a vegetarian consumes three times as much folic acid as an omnivore, however, the vegan diet does not provide enough vitamin B^{12}. It is wise to eat vitamin B^{12}-

fortified cereals and foods. Vegan diets can also be quite low in zinc and creatine and these may need to be supplemented. Finally, the omega-3 fatty acid found in vegan diets, alpha linolenic acid, is not efficiently used by humans and may increase the risk of prostate cancer. Vegans would probably benefit from supplementary DHA, the omega-3 fat found in fish. Fortunately, DHA from algae is now available in supplement form and is also used in most pediatric formulas.

Soy products are a good source of high-quality protein, iron, vitamins, and minerals. You can incorporate soy products into your diet in many different ways: try eating soybeans, tempeh, and tofu, for example. Tofu is very easy to cook or bake and comes in extra firm, firm, soft, and Silken form and can be marinated or baked. You should avoid fried tofu; frying causes dangerous changes to develop in the proteins. Extra firm and firm tofu are excellent for grilling, marinating, or cutting large chunks to use in stir-fry meals. Soft tofu is great for sauces, gravies, dips, and pasta fillings. Silken tofu is wonderful in dessert recipes, milk shakes, and creamy soups. Although tofu is cholesterol-free and low in saturated fat, it is high in total fat. This should not be of great concern because if you follow the diet we suggest, your total fat intake should be in balance. Olive oil is the only oil you will need because unsaturated is believed to be cancer-neutral. When using olive oil do not over heat it.

The Bottom Line

Here's our bottom line on what to eat and what to avoid:

· Eat plenty of fresh fruits and vegetables;

· Consume fiber;

· Totally eliminate all red meat;

· Limit animal products to skinless white meat of chicken or turkey, wild-caught fish, and shellfish;

· Combine rice or grains with legumes and other fresh vegetables to ensure proper nutrition;

· Balance protein, fats, and carbohydrates (30% good fats, 30% protein, 40% carbohydrates.)

CHAPTER 11

Cooking 101

Equipping Your Kitchen

A well-equipped kitchen makes cooking chores easier and more efficient. Having the right tool for the right job saves time and frustration. Our equipment includes the following:

Blender
Crock-Pot/Slow Cooker
Electric Mixer
Food Processor
Rice/Vegetable Steamer
Spice Grinder
Glass Canning Jars (1/2 pints, pints, quarts, 1/2 gallons)
Ice Cube Trays, Large and Small
Ramekins
Mortar & Pestle
Ricer (to hand-puree vegetables)
Wooden Cutting Boards
Wooden Spoons
A Wide Selection of Knives
Colanders
Garlic Presses
Ladles
Mushroom Brush
Pepper Mill
Pressure Cooker
Strainers
Vegetable Peeler
Whisk
Stainless Steel Pots and Pans

Juicer
Glass Jars and Storage Containers (avoid plastics)
Wax Paper (use plastic wrap sparingly—never heat plastic wrap)
Parchment Paper (unbleached)
Aluminum Foil

Stocking Your Kitchen

Our kitchens hold a variety of foods and staples used throughout this cookbook. We find that having these items on hand saves time and multiple shopping trips. You can also trim expenses by buying in quantity.

Pasta

Flavors Available:
　Whole wheat
　Spinach
　Tomato
　Lemon
Gluten-free pasta alternatives:
　Quinoa
　Brown Rice
　Corn
Various Shapes:
　Acine di Pepe
　Capellini (Angel Hair)
　Ditalini
　Farfalle
　Fettuccini
　Fusilli
　Linguini
　Orzo
　Penne
　Rigatoni
　Spaghetti
　Ziti

Rice

Arborio
Basmati (white and brown)
Brown, short/long grain
Risotto
White Jasmine
Wild

Grains

Barley
Buckwheat
Buglur
Farro
Groats
Job's Tears
Kamut
Kasha
Millet
Oats
Quinoa
Rye
Rye Berries
Wheat Berries

Peas

Green and yellow

Beans

Adzuki
Black
Black Turtle
Black-eyed Peas
Black Soybeans
Butter
Cannellini

Fava beans
Flageolet
Garbanzo beans
Great northern beans
Kidney
Lentils
>   Brown
>
>   Black
>
>   Green
>
>   Red
>
>   Yellow

Lima
Navy
Pinto
Soy

Herbs and Spices

Whenever possible, we use fresh herbs and spices. The vibrancy of just-plucked basil, oregano, thyme, and bay leaf can't be matched by their dried versions; fresh herbs and spices are healthier and more pungent, as well. However, sometimes you can only find a specific herb or spice dried, and in that case, use what you can find.

Allspice
Anise seed
Basil
Bay leaf
Black pepper
Caraway seed
Cardamom
Cayenne pepper
Celery seed
Chili powder
Cinnamon

Cloves
Coriander
Cumin, ground and seeds
Dill
Fennel
Fenugreek
Garam masala
Garlic
Ginger
Lemon rind
Orange rind
Marjoram
Mustard, ground and seeds
Nutmeg
Oregano
Parsley
Paprika
Poppy seed
Red pepper flakes
Rosemary
Saffron
Sage
Salt
Savory
Tarragon
Thyme
Turmeric

Vinegars

Balsamic (white/dark)
Cider
Champagne, white, and red wine

Favored Fat Sources and Oils

For a complete explanation of why we selected these fats and avoided others, please read the previous chapter.

Olives and olive oil
Almonds and almond oil
Pistachios
Hazelnuts and hazelnut oil
Cashews
Macadamia nuts
Avocado and avocado oil

Types of Olive Oil

Extra Virgin: extracted from olives on the first pressing, cold pressed without the use of heat or chemicals, it has a pure fruity taste and a golden to pale green hue. It is usually used as a flavoring and should not be subjected to heat.

Virgin: extracted from olives on the second pressing, and cold pressed also.

Olive oil: fits neither of the two descriptions above. Heat is usually used to extract the last bit of oil from the olives. This type is usually used for cooking over heat.

Where to Shop

In the United States, we are fortunate to have grocery markets that offer organically grown foods as well as those that are traditionally grown and raised. Many stores carry a good variety of fresh vegetables, fruits, herbs, fish, and meats. Larger markets have beans, whole grains, and a large variety of rice and pasta. In many areas there are small ethnic grocery markets and natural health food stores from which to supply your kitchen. You should always choose stores that rotate their stock frequently to obtain the freshest ingredients. Always check the dates! Whenever possible, buy fresh fruits, vegetables, meats, eggs, and grains from local farmers' markets; these products tend to be fresher than those stocked in supermarkets, as they are grown close to where they are sold.

Frozen foods

If you have difficulty obtaining fresh produce at certain times of the year, frozen foods are an excellent alternative because they are picked at the height of their freshness, quickly blanched, and flash-frozen. You may wish to add small amounts of frozen vegetables to your recipes.

Storing Grains & Beans

Store grains and beans in tightly-lidded glass jars. Mason or Bell jars in pints, quarts, and half gallons are very useful. We often save glass jars with good lids. We prefer glass because we can seal them tightly and odors are not picked up in the refrigerator. We use them in our cupboards and in the freezer too. Another advantage is that we can see exactly what and how much is in each jar. Labels attach and come off easily when we need to change them.

To use glass jars in the freezer fill the jar within an inch and a half from the top. Place the jar in the freezer on an angle. When the content is frozen seal with the lid.

Cooking Shortcuts & Tips

Here are some timesaving suggestions to make your cooking life easier.

Garlic

In our recipes we use a lot of garlic in the Mediterranean tradition. While peeling garlic cloves and using them immediately helps retain their full flavor and zing, you can peel two whole heads of garlic at a time and store them in a tightly-lidded glass jar. The cloves will keep in the refrigerator for up to two weeks. We like to avoid bags of pre-peeled cloves, because often the garlic is treated before it is bagged.

Olive Oil

Olive oil can be expensive in small quantities. We prefer to buy olive oil in 1/2 gallon or gallon containers. These containers can be hard to handle. Therefore, we pour the oil into small tightly sealed glass bottles. It is best to store them away from light.

Tofu

Tofu takes on the flavor of anything in which you marinate or cook it. To drain extra liquid from the tofu, place tofu between two plates and squeeze over the sink. If time permits, put a plate with a heavy object over the tofu in a shallow bowl. Let it sit for 30 minutes and then drain the excess liquid. To slice, set the tofu on a cutting board and use a serrated knife to cut slices to the desired size.

Rice & Beans

When we cook rice or beans, we make a little extra to use in lunches or in the next days' meals. On our day off, we will make a big batch of bean or grain-based soup, and rely on this soup for easy and healthy lunches during the workweek. We store these cooked portions in tightly-lidded containers in our refrigerator.

Vegetables

Instead of discarding the end pieces or vegetables close to the end of their shelf life, put them in a pot of water and simmer to make stock. Remove the vegetables and throw them away. Pour the cool stock into ice cube trays to freeze. Once frozen, store the cubes in Mason Jars. When you need a little bit of stock, it will be handy.

Breadcrumbs

When you have stale bread of any description, don't throw it away. Get out your food processor, toss in the bread, add a little chopped parsley, pulse, remove, and store in tightly-lidded glass jars.

Canned Beans

Some of the recipes in this cookbook use canned beans. We understand that when life gets busy, you might not have time to soak and cook beans. If you do purchase canned beans, make sure they are packaged in a BPA-free can. Currently, only one manufacturer uses BPA-free cans, Eden Organics. We hope that other manufactures will begin producing BPA-free cans soon, but in the meantime, we recommend purchasing the Eden Organics brand.

Cooking Beans

When we first started to cook and enjoy beans and grains, we had a difficult time finding soaking and cooking charts. We have assembled a guide to make this process easier for you.

It is important to rinse and visually inspect all rice, grains, and beans. Look for small rocks and debris like twigs that sometimes get mixed in with the product.

Season the grains, beans, and rice to your taste. We like to add a bay leaf, a halved yellow onion, and some herbs to the cooking liquid. Try replacing the cooking water with vegetable or chicken stock.

Whenever we cook grains and rice, we add a few pinches of salt to the cooking liquid. Many chefs are actually divided on when to season beans with salt; some adamantly claim that cooking beans in salted water makes the outer skin tough; others claim that the beans have no flavor and never taste seasoned if salt is added at the end of the cooking process. We find it helpful to lightly season the cooking liquid, and once the beans have cooked through, we add more salt and season the beans to our liking; this process yields a well-seasoned and creamy bean that can be used in any recipe.

Soaking reduces cooking time. If you do not soak the beans

they must be cooked 1/2 hour to 1 hour longer. Soaking the beans releases the gas-producing sugars into the soaking water, reducing the problem of flatulence. Soak most beans overnight, and change the water at least once. Replace water as needed, so the beans are always covered with liquid. Small beans will be softened in approximately 4 hours. Make sure to discard the soaking water. In the following instructions reduce the liquid by 1 part if you have soaked the beans before cooking. Bean cooking times vary depending on how long the batch has been dried, so check them about a 1/2 hour before the minimum time requirement. If they are not cooked yet, continue checking every 10 minutes or so.

Adzuki (aduke or auzki)
Adzuki are small brownish red beans with white stripes. These beans are a good source of vitamin B, calcium, and vitamin C, and are highly digestible. Use 3 cups of liquid to 1 cup of beans. Bring to a boil, reduce heat, and cover pan. Simmer for 1-1/2 to 2 hours.

Black Turtle Beans
These earthy, sweet tasting beans make superb soup. Use 3 cups liquid to 1 cup beans. Bring to a boil, reduce heat, cover, and simmer for 1-1/2 to 2 hours.

Black-eyed Peas
Black-eyed Peas were probably introduced to the United States by slaves from Africa. These beans are relatively quick cooking and require no presoaking. Use 3 cups water to 1 cup beans. Bring to a boil, reduce heat, cover, and simmer for 1/2 hour.

Black Soybeans
Black soybeans are available at most health food stores. They are round and plump with a glossy skin and are an excellent source of high quality protein. Use 3 cups water to 1 cup beans.

Bring to a boil, reduce heat, cover pot, and simmer for 2-3 hours.

Cannellini

These white, oval shaped beans are a favorite in Italy where they're the bean of choice for *pasta e fagioli*. Use 3 cups water to 1 cup beans. Bring to a boil, reduce heat, cover, and simmer for 1 to 1-1/2 hours.

Fava Beans

These beans are not readily available fresh in this country. The dried beans have a rusty brown colored skin; this tough skin must be peeled. Fava beans are wonderful pureed with a generous amount of olive oil and garlic. Use 3 cups of water to 1 cup of beans. Bring to a boil, reduce heat, cover pot, and simmer for 1-1/2 to 2 hours.

Flageolets

Flageolets are a favorite in France. They are pale green in color, hard to find fresh, and expensive. Use 3 cups water to 1 cup beans. Bring to a boil, reduce heat, cover pot, and simmer for 1 to 1-1/2 hours. Serve with a drizzle of extra virgin olive oil.

Garbanzo (Chickpeas, Ceci)

Chickpeas are round, bumpy, and beige with a nutty flavor and creamy texture. They are easy to puree and make excellent dips and spreads. Hummus is made from pureeing chickpeas with olive oil, lemon juice, garlic, tahini, and salt. To cook chickpeas, use 3 cups of water to 1 cup of beans. Bring the chickpeas to a boil, reduce the heat, cover the pot, and simmer for 1-1/2 to 2 hours.

Great Northern

These large white beans are grown in the Mid-western part of the United States. They hold up well to cooking and have a very mild flavor. Use 3 cups water to 1 cup beans. Bring to a boil, reduce heat, cover pot, and simmer for 1 to 1-1/2 hours.

Kidney

Kidney beans come in a variety of colors. Dark red kidney beans are the most widely used in American cooking. This bean is used in red beans and rice. And where would good old chili be without kidney beans? Use 3 cups of water to 1 cup of beans. Bring to a boil, reduce heat, cover pot, and simmer for 1-1/2 to 2 hours.

Lentils

An ancient legume and member of the pea family, lentils come in the following varieties: brown, green, red, yellow, and black. Lentils are high in protein and make a very good compliment to brown rice. Lentils do not require soaking. Use 3 cups of liquid to 1 cup of lentils. Bring the lentils to a boil, reduce the heat, cover the pot, and simmer for 20-40 minutes. Be careful not to overcook the lentils or they will become mushy.

Navy

Creamy, oval shaped beans are the best for baked beans. They're also ideal for purees. Use 3 cups of liquid to 1 cup of beans. Bring to a boil, reduce heat, cover pot, and simmer for 1-1/2 to 2 hours.

Pinto

These beans are often used in Mexican dishes like burritos, refried beans, and quesadillas. Use 3 cups liquid to 1 cup beans. Bring to a boil, reduce heat, cover pot, and simmer for 1-1/2 to 2 hours.

Scarlet Runner

Scarlet Runners are broad flat green pods with red seeds. You can eat the fresh whole bean or the dried inner seed. Use 3 cups liquid to 1 cup beans. Bring to a boil, reduce heat, cover pot, and simmer for 1-1/2 to 2 hours.

Soybeans

They are usually processed into tofu, tempeh, and soy sauce. Use 3 cups of liquid to 1 cup of beans. Bring to a boil, reduce heat, cover pot, and simmer for 2-3 hours.

Cooking Grains

When combined with beans, grains make a complete protein. They're also a delicious component to many of our recipes. Here's a guide to common and hard-to-find grains and tips on how to cook them.

Barley

Barley has a sweet mellow taste and a chewy texture and provides a substantial amount of fiber and minerals. It expands in cooking: 1 cup of dry will produce 3-4 cups cooked. Use 2 parts liquid to 1 part barley; bring to a boil, cover, reduce heat, and simmer for 40 minutes. Let stand, covered, for 7 minutes.

Couscous

A staple of North Africa, couscous is made from durum wheat stripped of its bran and germ. A whole-wheat couscous is distributed by Neshamany Valley. It is brown rather than cream-colored because it is made from the whole grain. Bring 2 cups of liquid to a boil. Whisk in 1 cup couscous, then cook for 1 minute while whisking continuously. Cover pot, turn off heat and let steam to absorb the liquid, about 10-15 minutes. Fluff with a fork.

Job's Tears

Job's tears looks like oversized pearl barley: it is light brown with an indented stripe running down the middle. They are chewy and release starch in cooking, which gives a slight stickiness to the grains. First lightly toast the grains in the oven on a baking sheet. Use 1 1/2 cups water to 1 cup of Job's tears. Bring to a boil, reduce heat, and simmer for 1 hour. Let stand for 5 minutes.

Kasha

Kasha is the commonly available form of buckwheat. Use 2 cups liquid to 1 cup Kasha. Bring to a boil, reduce heat, and watch very closely until liquid is all but absorbed. Immediately remove from heat. Cover and let the grains stand until the remaining liquid is absorbed.

Millet

Millet is a nutritional giant with a generous protein profile and large amounts of B vitamins, iron, potassium, magnesium, and phosphorus. It is easier to digest than many other grains. It stands up well to strong flavors. Use 2-1/2 cups liquid to 1 cup millet. Bring to a boil and reduce heat. Cover the pan and gently simmer the millet for 40 minutes. The grains should be fluffy when you remove the lid.

Quinoa

Native to the Andes, quinoa is about the size of sesame seeds. Quinoa has a more impressive protein profile than wheat and contains numerous amino acids. Right now there are three varieties of quinoa available in the United States: white/beige, red, and the harder to find black. Lightly toast the quinoa in a little olive oil. Add 2 cups water to 1 cup quinoa, bring to a boil, reduce heat to low, cover, and simmer until all liquid is absorbed. Grains will appear fluffy. Quinoa is easy to overcook; we find it best to take it off the heat when there is still a slight bite to the grain. Overcooked quinoa tends to be mushy and water-loaded.

Basmati Rice

Authentic basmati is imported from India or Pakistan. It has a nutty aroma and a chewy texture. Use 2 cups liquid to 1 cup rice. Boil water and add rice. Stir and let boil again. Reduce heat, cover, and simmer for 25 minutes. Let stand for 5 minutes and then fluff with a fork.

Brown Rice

Nutritionally more complete because it has not been stripped of its hull, bran, and germ. It can be either short or long grained. Long grain is less chewy and fluffier than the short grain. Use 2 cups liquid to 1 cup brown rice. Bring liquid to a boil and stir in rice. Reduce heat after a minute and simmer, covered, for 40 minutes. Do not remove lid for 10 minutes after removal from the heat. The trapped steam will plump the grains.

Wild Rice

Wild rice is not really rice, but seeds of a native North American aquatic grass. Wild rice is high in protein and a good source of vitamin B. Use 3 to 4 cups liquid to 1 cup wild rice. Bring liquid to a boil and stir in rice, reduce heat, cover tightly, and simmer for 45 minutes. Drain remaining liquid and let stand covered for 5 minutes. Fluff with a fork. One cup of wild rice yields about 4 cups cooked rice.

Wehani Rice

This mahogany-colored whole grain rice has a nutty flavor and is chewy in texture. Use 2-1/2 cups liquid to 1 cup Wehani rice. Bring liquid and rice to a boil, reduce heat, cover and simmer for 45 minutes. Do not remove the lid, turn heat off and allow to sit covered for 15 minutes.

Wheat Berries

Cooked berries are always chewy, even when thoroughly cooked. Use 4 cups of liquid to 1 cup of wheat berries. Bring to a boil, immediately reduce heat, and simmer for 1-1/2 hours.

CHAPTER 12
Traditional Soy Products

Soy products are a good source of protein and genistein. In addition to boosting protein in any dish, they are a good way to add variety to your cooking. Many soy products take on the flavor of the spices in which they are cooked.

Here are some common soy products:

Roasted Soybeans
Soybeans can be roasted in the oven or heated in a skillet. The browned soybeans are then commonly salted. You can eat them just as you would peanuts. To minimize fat content, we recommend that you use dry roasted beans.

Green Soybeans
These are specific strains of soybeans that are best eaten as you would lima beans. They must be cooked to avoid the toxins in the uncooked bean. Just steam or boil them in salted water while still in the pod. They can be eaten hot or chilled and used in any dish that calls for lima beans. The Japanese call these salted steamed beans Edamame. The fresh green soybeans are available in many Asian grocery stores. Out of season, we have found them in the frozen food sections. If you have a vegetable garden, they are easy to grow. Seeds are available from Park Seeds and Johnny's Select Seeds. Our current favorite is the Butterbean variety from Johnny's Select Seeds. Green soybeans can be grown in northern areas where limas do not do as well.

Black Soybeans
The usual soybeans found in health food stores are pale brown or beige. These are used in most of the recipes you might

encounter. There are also black soybeans, which are well worth the search. Their skin is thinner, they cook more rapidly, and we find their flavor very appealing. They can readily be incorporated into many bean dishes.

Soy Flour

We prefer Japanese-style soy flour simply made from ground soybeans. This flour is used to make soymilk and tofu. Our favorite is soy flour that has been toasted. In the European cooking tradition, browning flour is a standard step in making gravy. We find that this browned soy flour serves very well as a substitute. However, this flour is not fat-free: about 40% of the calories come from fat.

Soymilk

This soy beverage is widely used in the United States as a basis for nondairy infant formulas. Most health food stores and upscale grocery stores carry soymilk formulated for adults and chain stores like Safeway carry the product as well. For example, in Charlottesville, Virginia, a town of less than 100,000, several brands of soymilk for adults are available. Soymilk comes plain, unsweetened, or flavored with vanilla or chocolate. While we think all varieties taste just fine, we prefer the unsweetened version. However, soymilk does not at all remind us of cow's milk. If you are really attached to the taste of cow's milk, you can mix soy milk with skim milk. Another alternative that yields a very rich tasting drink is adding fat-free, dried instant milk to soymilk. Our favorite recipe is to put soymilk into a blender and add frozen strawberries, raspberries or blueberries until the mixture is too thick for the blender to stir. We add some sugar and, at times, ginger to this mixture.

Tempeh

Tempeh is made by combining soybeans with grains, such as barley or rice and then letting them ferment for a very short period of time. The end result is a firm slab. When cooked, tempeh has a meaty and nutty flavor. Baking or lightly sautéing the product yields fantastic results. When it has browned, we place it on a bun with mustard and onions. We also dice it into small cubes and add it to soups, stews, or spaghetti sauce.

Tofu

Tofu was first used in China some time around 200 B.C. According to the Soyfoods Association of America, the discovery of the process is lost to the ages. Ancient Chinese legend says that the first tofu was created by accident. A cook added nigari, a compound found in natural ocean water, to flavor pureed cooked soybeans and that produced the curd that we know today as tofu. Tofu is a dietary staple throughout Asia. It is made fresh daily in thousands of small tofu shops and sold in the street. Tofu acts like a sponge in recipes, absorbing the flavor of anything that it is added to.

Tofu is made from soymilk by a process very similar to that used to make cheese from cow's milk. Calcium and other compounds are added to the soymilk to cause it to coagulate. The coagulated soymilk is then placed in wooden or stainless steel molds and excess water allowed to drain away.

Tofu is very bland in taste, but will take on the taste of whatever it is cooked in. It can be diced and mixed easily with soups or stews. We find it mixes well in the tomato sauce we use for spaghetti as well as in the smoothie recipe we discussed above.

Rich in high-quality protein, tofu is an excellent source of B vitamins and iron. When the curdling agent used to make tofu is a calcium salt, the tofu is a good source of calcium. Fifty percent of the calories in tofu come from fat. However, a four-ounce serving contains just 6 grams of fat. It is low in saturated fat and contains no cholesterol. Generally the softer the tofu, the lower the fat content. Tofu is also very low in sodium, making it a perfect food for people on sodium-restricted diets.

Recipes

Vinaigrettes
& Sauces

Balsamic & Herb Vinaigrette

This recipe pairs fresh herbs with sweet Balsamic vinegar. Bitter greens in the chicory family (radicchio, endive, frisée, and dandelion), become even more delicious when offset by Balsamic's sweet acidity.

SHOPPING LIST
1/3 cup of Balsamic vinegar
1/2 cup of extra virgin olive oil
2-3 peeled and minced garlic cloves
1/2 teaspoon fresh or dried basil
1/2 teaspoon fresh or dried oregano
Salt and black pepper, to taste

PREPARATION
Place all the ingredients in a bottle. Cork or twist shut, and shake thoroughly. Let the vinaigrette stand for five minutes. Shake again right before serving over salad greens.

Prep time 12 minutes.

Serves 6-8.

Notes

Mustard Garlic Vinaigrette

This easy-to-assemble vinaigrette combines mustard's kick with the intensity of fresh minced garlic. If uncooked garlic tends to overwhelm you, try macerating it in champagne vinegar and mustard for 30 minutes before whisking in the olive oil. Try this vinaigrette with tender spinach leaves, which contain high levels of lutein, an antioxidant that protects the eyes from macular degeneration and has some anticancer activity.

SHOPPING LIST
1 tablespoon Dijon mustard
1-2 garlic cloves, minced
3 tablespoons extra virgin olive oil
1 tablespoon champagne vinegar
Salt and black pepper, to taste

PREPARATION
In a small bowl combine the ingredients. Mix thoroughly with a whisk. Add the mixture to leaves of romaine or spinach and toss thoroughly to coat. The recipe can be doubled or tripled for larger salads.

Prep time 10 minutes.

Serves 1-2.

Variations Add 1 teaspoon of honey to the vinaigrette, or dried cranberries and slivered almonds to the salad.

Notes

Red Wine Shallot Vinaigrette

The method included in this recipe allows you to create emulsified vinaigrette in three easy steps.

SHOPPING LIST
1/3 cup red wine vinegar
1/2 cup extra virgin olive oil
2 medium shallots, minced
Salt and black pepper, to taste

PREPARATION
Place all the ingredients in a bottle. Cork or twist shut, and shake thoroughly. Let the vinaigrette stand for five minutes. Shake again right before serving over salad greens.

Prep time 5 minutes.

Serves 6-8.

Notes

Fresh Dill and Shallot Vinaigrette

Fresh dill and shallots make this bright vinaigrette visually appealing. Try mixing this dressing with an iceberg, frisée, or endive salad.

SHOPPING LIST
1/3 cup rice vinegar
1/2 cup extra virgin olive oil
1 teaspoon Dijon mustard
2 small shallots, minced
1 tablespoon fresh dill, chopped
Salt, to taste

PREPARATION
In a small bowl combine the ingredients and whisk for 1 minute. Add the vinaigrette to salad greens or cooked vegetables. Store the vinaigrette in a tightly lidded glass jar and refrigerate. Keeps for 2 – 3 weeks without fresh dill; add dill before serving to avoid browning.

Prep time 5 minutes.

Serves 6-8.

Notes

Indian Curry Vinaigrette

This vinaigrette uses curry powder and cumin to create an intense and unexpected twist on the common salad dressing. Curry powder contains turmeric, a tasty antioxidant. Try it mixed with spinach and sliced apple for a super-food salad.

SHOPPING LIST
3 tablespoons rice vinegar
2 tablespoons apple juice
3 tablespoons hazelnut or extra virgin olive oil
2 teaspoons stone ground mustard
1 teaspoon soy sauce
1/2 teaspoon curry powder
1/8 teaspoon black pepper
1/8 teaspoon cumin
Salt, to taste

PREPARATION
Whisk the vinegar, apple juice, soy sauce, mustard, herbs, and spices in a small bowl. Slowly whisk in the olive oil. Add the mixture to salad greens.

Prep time 5 minutes.

Serves 6-8.

Notes

Sweet and Sour Dressing

Try this dressing with endive leaves or other mildly bitter greens like radicchio or arugula.

SHOPPING LIST
1 tablespoon lemon juice
2 tablespoons olive oil
1 teaspoon honey
1/4 cup mint, chopped
Salt, to taste

PREPARATION
Whisk the ingredients in a small bowl, and toss your favorite salad greens with the dressing.

Prep time 5 minutes.

Serves 1-2.

Notes

Raspberry Vinaigrette

This vinaigrette adds striking color and flavor to any salad. In the summer months, when you can find fresh raspberries and herbs, raspberry vinaigrette becomes an easy way to incorporate more red fruit into your diet. If you can find good frozen raspberries, make sure to thaw the fruit before adding it to the blender.

SHOPPING LIST
1/2 cup raspberries
1/4 cup extra virgin olive oil
1/4 cup raspberry vinegar
1 small shallot
1/4 teaspoon sugar
Ground black pepper and salt, to taste

PREPARATION
Put all the ingredients in a blender and puree until smooth. Let the vinaigrette stand for one hour and pour it over greens of your choice. If you don't use all the dressing store it in the refrigerator.

Prep time 5 minutes. *Total time* 1 hour.

Serves 4-6.

Notes

Apple Cider Vinaigrette

Try apple cider vinaigrette with crispy iceberg lettuce, thin slices of fresh apples, and roasted and chopped hazelnuts.

SHOPPING LIST
1/4 cup apple cider vinegar
2 tablespoons apple juice
1/2 cup extra virgin olive oil
1/8 teaspoon black pepper
Salt, to taste

PREPARATION
Whisk together the vinegar and apple juice. Season the mix generously with salt and pepper. Slowly whisk in the olive oil, adjust the seasoning, and serve.

Prep time 5 minutes. *Total time* 1 hour.

Serves 4-6.

Notes

Ginger Lemon Soy Sauce

Fresh grated ginger suppresses inflammation and nausea and has anticancer activity. Combining ginger with lemon juice makes this savory dressing a great alternative to heavy dressings like blue cheese or ranch.

SHOPPING LIST
3-1/2 tablespoons soy sauce
2 tablespoons lemon juice
3-4 tablespoons olive oil
1 teaspoon freshly grated ginger

PREPARATION
Combine and mix all the ingredients. Let stand for 15-20 minutes. Toss with either fresh salad greens or pour over an assortment of cooked vegetables.

Prep time 5 minutes.

Serves 4-8.

Notes

Lemon, Garlic, and Mint Salsa

This piquant mix works well to brighten chicken and potato salads, and acts as a great substitute for the traditional mustard and mayonnaise combination.

SHOPPING LIST
1/4 cup lemon juice
1/2 cup extra virgin olive oil
2 garlic cloves, minced
2 tablespoon fresh mint, minced
2 tablespoons lemon zest
1/8 teaspoon white pepper
Salt, to taste

PREPARATION
Mix together all ingredients except the lemon juice. Make sure to coat the mint in the olive oil to prevent oxidation. Right before serving, mix in the lemon juice, and adjust seasoning to taste. You can toss this sauce with torn cooked chicken breast or roasted potatoes for a healthy chicken or potato salad.

Prep time 5 minutes.

Serves 4-6.

Notes

Lemon Vinaigrette

This basic vinaigrette highlights lemon's unique flavor by incorporating zest into the base. Try lemon vinaigrette over shredded vegetable salads or with almost any green salad. Please note that lemons vary in acidity, so you may need to adjust the amount of olive oil you add.

SHOPPING LIST
1 lemon, zested
1/4 cup lemon juice
1–1-1/4 cup extra virgin olive oil
1-1/2 teaspoons sugar (optional)
Salt, to taste

PREPARATION
In a large bowl, mix the zest, lemon juice, sugar, and salt; let the ingredients sit for ten minutes before slowly whisking in the olive oil. Adjust the seasoning to taste, and serve or store refrigerated in an airtight container.

Prep Time 5 minutes. *Total Time* 15 minutes.

Serves 4-6.

Notes

Spicy Mango Condiment

Mangos are now widely available in North American supermarkets; their tang compliments a variety of savory dishes. Although many Americans have eaten mangos as a raw fruit, most do not know how good they can be when cooked. The following recipe makes a fruit sauce similar to an Indian chutney, which is commonly used as a condiment for lentil, rice, and meat dishes. Try this sauce on seared fish and grilled poultry. The intense flavors bloom when spread on toasted sourdough bread.

SHOPPING LIST
4 ripe mangos
1-2 ounces Jalapeno (or Poblano if you like mild spice)
6 garlic cloves
1 tablespoon extra virgin olive oil
2 tablespoons rice wine vinegar
1/4 cup brown sugar
1/2 cup raisins (*optional*)
2 tablespoons orange or lemon zest
Salt, to taste

PREPARATION
Garlic: Peel and crush.

Jalapeno/Poblano Wearing latex gloves (trust us)
Wash and dry, remove vein and seed, then mince. Simmer peppers in vinegar.

Mangos
Wash and dry, peel off skin and discard, then trim the flesh from the stone. Chop fruit flesh into 1/2 inch chunks.

Cook the jalapenos in the vinegar as stated above. In a separate pan, bloom the garlic in olive oil. Then place the mango, garlic, brown sugar, lemon or orange zest, and jalapenos in a heavy bottom saucepan and simmer until the mangoes are soft; no more than five minutes. Add optional raisins before cooking. Once the sauce has cooled, refrigerate it for an hour or more to allow the flavors to mingle. Serve warm or cold.

Prep time 30 minutes. *Total time* 1-1/2 hours.

Serves 8.

Notes

Pistachio and Basil Pesto

This cheese-free version of traditional pesto uses pistachios to mimic the richness of Parmesan. While great mixed into pasta, this sauce also works well drizzled over vegetables such as carrots or cauliflower, as a spread for sandwiches, or simply stirred into soups.

SHOPPING LIST
3 tablespoons pistachios, roasted
4 cups packed (or two bunches), picked and washed fresh
   basil leaves
1 lemon, zested
5 cloves garlic, minced
6 ounces extra virgin olive oil
Salt, to taste

PREPARATION
Make sure to wash and thoroughly dry the basil leaves. Place all the ingredients in a blender, adding the oil last. You may need to blend the basil leaves in batches—just blend and add until all leaves are incorporated into the mixture. Blend until smooth. Store pesto in an airtight container. If you need to store it for a few days, make sure there is a thin layer of oil on the top to prevent oxidation. Alternatively, you might want to place a piece of plastic wrap pressed into the mixture to seal it from the air.

Prep Time 25-35 minutes.

Serves 4-6.

Notes

Aioli

One of the most versatile sauces, aioli can be dolloped over chicken, fish, or vegetables, used to help bind crab cakes, swirled into clear soups, or lathered onto sandwich bread. From the aioli base, you can add chopped or pureed herbs, cornichons, diced shallots, paprika, or a host of other ingredients to create a sauce to fit any dish. We think it is important to know how to make this sauce, which can substitute for the mayonnaise so readily available at most grocery stores. You will want to avoid the canola-based mayonnaise that comes on your store shelves. This olive oil-based alternative provides healthful benefits while allowing you to indulge in the unctuous.

SHOPPING LIST
3-4 cloves of garlic
1 lemon, juiced
Salt
2 large egg yolks
1-1/2 cups light olive oil

PREPARATION
Whisk method: Place the garlic cloves and salt in a mortar. Grind and pound the garlic until it forms a smooth paste. Squeeze the lemon in the mortar with the garlic, and stir. Dump the garlic lemon mixture into a stainless steel bowl and add the egg yolks. Immediately whisk the yolks into the garlic and lemon until slightly frothy. Very slowly (drop by drop!) add the olive oil to the bowl, while vigorously whisking the mixture. The key to an unbroken sauce is to go slow for the first 3/4 of a cup of oil; once you emulsify 3/4 cup, you can add the oil a *little* faster. Keep whisking! When all the oil is emulsified, taste the mixture and adjust the seasoning with salt and lemon juice.

Food processor method: While hand-whisking aioli creates a divinely light and airy texture, the method does take some time, and often time is what we lack. If you are in a hurry, the following method should work well. Repeat the first few steps of mortaring the garlic and salt until smooth and add the lemon juice, but instead of placing the mixture in a bowl, place it in the food processor. With the blade running, slowly (drop by drop!) add the olive oil. Once you have emulsified about 3/4 to 1 cup of the oil, you can begin to add it at a faster rate. Do not dump all the oil in though, still take your time and allow each drizzle of oil to emulsify before continuing. When all the oil is suspended in the mixture, stop the processor. If you over-process the sauce it will break. Season the aioli to taste with salt and lemon juice.

If the aioli is too stiff, simply whisk in a drop or two of water to loosen the sauce.

Prep Time 10-15 Minutes.

Serves 4-8 (the serving yield depends on how you use the aioli).

Notes

Rapini, Garlic, and Hot Pepper

On cold winter days this dish will warm you with spicy and nourishing hot pepper, rapini and garlic. Mix into a pasta that can catch the textures of the sauce, such as conchiglie, corkscrew, or farfalle. Try the hot greens on grilled toast for a fantastic appetizer. You can substitute black or curly kale if you cannot find rapini, or do not like the green's slight bitterness.

SHOPPING LIST
1 bunch, rapini (or 1-1/2 cups of cooked rapini)
1 lemon, zested
4 cloves garlic, minced
1/4 cup extra-virgin olive oil
1/2 teaspoon red pepper flakes
1/8 teaspoon ground black pepper
Parmesan grated over the top of the pasta
1/8 teaspoon ground black pepper
Salt, to taste

PREPARATION
Bring a large pot of salted water to boil. Check for and remove any tough stems from the rapini. Place the rapini into the boiling water. Cook until slightly tender. Rapini cooks quickly, and should take no more than 2 minutes (of course this depends on the maturity of the rapini you have purchased). Pull the rapini out of the water with a strainer, or use a colander in your sink to drain. Spread the greens on a plate or a sheet tray to cool. Once the rapini is cool, chop it up into 1/2 inch chunks. In a saucepan over low heat, add your olive oil, garlic, and hot and black peppers. As the garlic begins to "bloom," or become fragrant and bubbles slightly, add the rapini and lemon zest to the pan and season with salt. Cook and stir the rapini into the oil until it is heated throughout. Remove from heat.

Stir into your favorite cooked pasta. If you can eat cheese, grate Parmesan or ricotta salata over the top to finish.

Prep Time 20 minutes.

Serves 4.

Notes

Mint Salsa Verde

This refreshing and intense sauce works well spooned over fish, chicken, or an assortment of roasted vegetables. Try substituting the mint with parsley for an equally delicious sauce that retains its vibrant green color.

SHOPPING LIST
2 bunches or 3 packed cups washed fresh mint leaves
3/4 cup extra-virgin olive oil
1/4 cup minced shallots
1/5 cup red wine vinegar
1 teaspoon chopped capers
Salt, to taste

PREPARATION
Make sure all water is dried from the washed mint leaves. Add the leaves and salt to the blender, then pour in olive oil. If you need to add the mint in batches, just blend it in until all the mint is incorporated. Spoon the mixture into a bowl. Stir in chopped capers. Mince the shallots, place in a small bowl, and submerge in red wine vinegar. Stir in a little salt, and let the shallots macerate for at least a half hour in the vinegar. Right before serving, mix the shallot-vinegar mixture into the mint-oil mixture. Mix in only what you will use for this meal; the shallots don't hold well in the sauce for more than a day. Taste for salt and acidic balance. Spoon the verde over roast chicken, fish, or grilled vegetables.

Prep Time 15-20 minutes.

Serves 4-6.

Notes

Green Olive and Orange Tapenade

The following tapenade can be made a day ahead and used on roasted or sautéed chicken and white fish. Try it on grilled or toasted bread for a healthy and rich snack. This tapenade also can serve as the base for a delicious pasta sauce. Simply add cooked artichokes or fresh tomatoes and toss into spaghettini or fettuccini. Castelvetrano olives are bright green and briny; if you cannot find these delicious olives, feel free to substitute with another green or black olive.

SHOPPING LIST
3/4 cup castelvetrano olives, chopped fine
1 teaspoon orange zest
1 teaspoon parsley
1 teaspoon balsamic vinegar
1 clove garlic, crushed into a paste
1/2 cup extra virgin olive oil
1 anchovy, chopped fine (Optional)

PREPARATION
Rinse, drain, and chop the olives. You may need to take a pairing knife and peel the flesh from the pit if the olives are not pitted already. Use a fine zester or microplane to zest a ripe orange. Finely chop parsley. Use the side of a large kitchen knife to crush and mash the garlic clove. Place all ingredients in a medium-sized stainless steel bowl, and stir to combine. Let the flavors blend for at least an hour before serving.

Prep Time 20-30 minutes.

Serves 4-6 (as a topping for chicken or fish)

Notes

Savory Split Green Peas

This hearty sauce tastes great over tempeh or tofu. You can also cool the mixture and use it as a spread on rice cakes or toast, or as a healthy and textured chip dip.

SHOPPING LIST
4-5 cloves garlic, chopped fine
1 medium onion, small dice
1 ounce olive oil
1/8 teaspoon red pepper flakes
1/8 tsp black pepper, ground
1/2 tsp whole caraway seeds, toasted
4 to 4 1/2 cups water
1 teaspoon lemon juice
1 cup split peas, dry

PREPARATION
Heat the olive oil in a large pot over medium heat. Add the onion, garlic, caraway, red pepper, black pepper, and salt. Sauté until the garlic and onions are translucent. Meanwhile, rinse the dry peas and sift for rocks or foreign material. Drain the peas, and add them to the pot. Stir to coat the peas with the oil and spices, and add the water. Bring the peas and liquid up to a light boil, reduce to a simmer, and cover. Cook until the peas are soft (but don't allow them to become a mass of mush). Dried beans and peas vary in their cooking times and the amount of water required, so you will have to taste the mixture, and adjust your cooking time and the amount of water appropriately. The amount of liquid left in the pot when the peas are cooked should be minimal, and the resulting sauce thick and tight. Finish the mixture with lemon juice. Depending on your taste, you might want to add a little extra virgin olive oil and parsley before serving.

Prep Time 50-70 minutes

Serves 3-4

Notes

Watercress Sauce

The following recipe is adapted from *The Slow Mediterranean Kitchen*, by Paula Wolfert. We've taken out the cream and lobster reduction for health reasons, but the resulting sauce is still rich and indulgent. The brilliant green color of this intense sauce works well with a variety of fatty fish from cod to salmon to fresh sardines.

SHOPPING LIST

3/4 cup rice milk (unsweetened, plain)
1-1/2 bunches fresh watercress
1 teaspoon lemon juice
1 teaspoon lemon zest
1/2 cube of vegetable bouillon
Salt and pepper to taste

PREPARATION
Rinse and drain the watercress. Pick off the large or tough stems with leggy roots. You should have about 2 cups of leaves and stems. Bring a large pot of water to boil. Season with salt as it cooks. On a low boil, cook the watercress for 10 minutes. Drain and place in an ice-bath until the watercress is cool. Squeeze the greens with your hands to drain as much water as possible. Place the watercress, 1/2 cup rice milk, 1/2 teaspoon salt, 1/4 teaspoon pepper, lemon zest, and 1/2 teaspoon of lemon juice in the blender. Puree until smooth. In a heavy saucepan, place the 1/2 cup of bouillon and 1/4 cup of unsweetened rice milk (please do not substitute with the regular sweetened rice milk, which contains quite a bit of sugar). Melt the bouillon into the milk over low heat. Whisk in the watercress puree. Adjust your seasoning, add lemon juice and salt if necessary. Serve the sauce hot.

Prep time 30 minutes

Serves 4-5

Spring Onion Relish With Lemon and Parsley

This relish pairs the spring onion's tender sweetness with the brightness of lemon-infused olive oil. These simple flavors are delicious when spread on grilled bread, nested on roasted halibut, or cresting a chicken's roasted breast. Please do not substitute scallions or green onions for real spring onions. Spring onions are young Torpedo, Walla Walla, red, or yellow onions before they set their bulbs. These tender onions might be harder to locate in the grocery store, so allow some leisure time at a farmers' market to find them.

SHOPPING LIST
1 bunch spring onions, trimmed of roots, cleaned, washed, and split in half
2 ounces white wine
1 ounce water
1 tablespoon olive oil
1 bay leaf
1 tablespoon lemon zest
1/2 cup Agrumato or lemon-infused olive oil
Salt to taste

PREPRATION
Preheat oven to 350°F. Place the split and cleaned onions in a roasting pan with wine, olive oil, salt, and bay leaf. Cover the roasting pan with parchment paper and then aluminum foil, and roast until tender, approximately 30-45 minutes. Remove from the oven, take off the foil, and let cool in the wine liquid. Once the onions have cooled, remove them from the liquid and slice or chop them into 1/4 inch slices. Place the onion in a bowl, and mix in 1 tablespoon of lemon zest, 1/2 cup Agrumato and a teaspoon of salt (according to taste). Chop 1/4 cup parsley, and stir into the onion relish. Let the relish sit for at least half an hour before serving to let the flavors develop.

Prep time 1 hour and 15 minutes.

Serves 4-6

Notes

Tomatillo Salsa

You can add cilantro to this salsa if you like. The sweet onions and garlic balance the tomatillo's piquancy. We love this sauce on tacos, burritos, nachos (baked chips, not fried), roasted fish, and chicken.

SHOPPING LIST
1 pound fresh tomatillos, dehusked and washed
1 medium onion, small dice
4 small garlic cloves, chopped fine
1 jalapeno, cut in half and cleaned of seeds
4 tablespoons olive oil
Salt and pepper to taste
1 ounce chopped cilantro (*Optional*)

PREPARATION
Preheat the oven to 400°F. Toss the halved and seedless jalapeno and the dehusked and washed tomatillos in a little olive oil and salt. Place the tomatillos and jalapeno in a roasting pan and cook until the skins blister slightly and the vegetables become soft (but not completely mushy). Set aside and let them cool enough to handle. Small dice the onion and fine chop the garlic cloves. Slightly heat the 4 tablespoons of olive oil in a sauté pan and add the onion and garlic. Slowly cook the onion and garlic until translucent. Season with salt and pepper. Once cool fine chop the jalapeno and rough chop the tomatillos, and add to the now translucent onion and garlic mixture. Continue cooking on a low-medium flame until the flavors blend and the vegetables break down a little, about 3- 5 minutes. Let the mixture cool to room temperature before adding chopped cilantro. Depending on the acidity of your tomatillos, you might want to add a small amount of fresh lime juice to brighten the salsa.

Prep time 1 hour

Serves 4-5

Notes

Salads

Summer Corn and Bean Salad

You can quickly assemble this salad for a potluck, BBQ, or spontaneous summer luncheon. If you have time, try roasting the corn in a hot oven; after roasting, scrape off the cob's tender kernels with a knife. The roasted corn adds a complexity of flavor that you cannot get from canned corn.

SHOPPING LIST

2 15-ounce cans black beans
1 15-ounce can chickpeas
   (also referred to as garbanzo or ceci beans)
1 green bell pepper diced
1 red bell pepper diced
3 plum tomatoes diced
1-1/2 cups cooked corn
3/4 cup chopped fresh cilantro
1 large finely chopped red onion
Salt, to taste

Vinaigrette
1 tablespoon apple cider vinegar
1/4 cup of lime juice
4 finely chopped garlic cloves
2 teaspoons cumin
1 teaspoon coriander
1/2 teaspoon freshly ground black pepper
1/2 cup extra virgin olive oil
Salt, to taste

PREPARATION

Drain and rinse the beans in cold water. In a large bowl combine the beans and the vegetables. In a small bowl whisk the vinaigrette ingredients until they form an emulsion. Pour the dressing over the vegetables and stir until all ingredients are coated with the vinaigrette.

Prep time 20-25 minutes.

Serves 8 – 10

Notes

Warm Cabbage With Apple and Hazelnuts

Red cabbage is available throughout the winter months, and this salad makes eating the antioxidant-rich vegetable fun and convenient. The vibrant colors of the acidified cabbage and onions provide unexpected cheeriness on a cold winter day. Do your best to find a recently harvested cabbage—while cabbage can store for several months, the difference in texture and taste between a fresh and month old cabbage is dramatic.

SHOPPING LIST
1 small red onion, thinly sliced
2 garlic cloves, minced
1 small red cabbage, thinly sliced (5-6 cups)
1 tart green apple, diced
1/4 cup Balsamic vinegar
1/2 cup extra virgin olive oil
2 tablespoons parsley, chopped
¼ cup hazelnuts, coarsely chopped
1 tablespoon apple cider vinegar
1/8 teaspoon black pepper
Salt, to taste

PREPARATION
Toast the hazelnuts in a 350°F, oven until aromatic. Let the nuts cool before chopping, and then set them aside in a small bowl. Heat the oil and balsamic vinegar in a large skillet. Add the onion and garlic and cook for three minutes on medium heat. Add the cabbage. Toss the cabbage in the oil and vinegar gently until it wilts and the color changes from purple to bright pink. Remove the pan from the heat; add the apple, hazelnuts, additional apple cider vinegar, parsley, and pepper. Stir and mix the salad right before serving.

Prep time 30 minutes.

Serves 6.

Notes

Radish, Lemon, and Mint Salad

The following recipe was developed at the suggestion of the late Laura Trent of Tip Top Produce. As the rains begin to subside in early spring in Northern California, radishes plump in the soil, lemons hang heavy on the trees, and tender sprigs of mint delicately leaf out. We find this salad refreshing on warm afternoons. Sliced radishes hold up well and develop in flavor over time; this dish is great for picnics or events in which the food needs to sit before it is eaten.

SHOPPING LIST
5 Watermelon Radishes, halved, then sliced into thin disks
3 cloves garlic, minced
2 lemons, 1 zested and segmented and 1 juiced
1/4 cup extra virgin olive oil
Sea salt, to taste
8 mint leaves, cut in very thin ribbons

PREPARATION
Juice 1 lemon and set aside. Zest the remaining lemon and segment it by dividing the meat from the pith of the fruit. Slice the segments with your knife so they are the size of a nickel. Mince the garlic, and add it to the reserved lemon juice with the zest and segments. Season this mixture well with salt. Allow the garlic and lemon to sit at room temperature for 20 minutes to allow the flavors to develop. Meanwhile, halve the watermelon radish, and slice them into paper-thin disks with your knife or a mandolin. Place the radish slices in a stainless-steel bowl. After 20 minutes, whisk the extra virgin olive oil into the garlic-lemon base. Pour this vinaigrette over the radishes, and toss the ingredients until the radish slices are coated with the vinaigrette. If necessary, adjust the seasoning with more salt. Slice thin ribbons of mint and fold it into the salad just before serving.

Prep Time 10 minutes. *Total time* 30 minutes.

Serves 4-6.

Notes

Red Bean and Onion Salad

This filling salad combines sweet red onions, nonfat mayo, and plump kidney beans to make a quick, but colorful lunch. Our dear friend Michael Forrest contributed this salad on a trip to our favorite summer spot, Smith Mountain Lake.

SHOPPING LIST
3 15-ounce cans red kidney beans
2 large red onions, diced
1/2 cup olive oil mayonnaise (or make your own aioli!)
1 teaspoon stone ground mustard
Ground black pepper and salt, to taste

PREPARATION
Drain the beans. In a small bowl, combine the mayonnaise, mustard, and pepper and whisk the ingredients together. In a large bowl, combine the beans and the onions. Add the dressing and toss together.

Prep time 15 minutes.

Serves 6.

Notes

Herbed Cucumber and Tomato Salad

Ripe cucumbers and tomatoes just picked from the vine, or culled from a farmer's flat, do not need extensive handling from any cook. The recipe below highlights the intense flavors of sun-ripened produce.

SHOPPING LIST
3 large cucumbers, peeled if waxed, deseeded, and sliced
2-3 large heirloom tomatoes, diced
1 teaspoon fresh basil, torn
1/2 teaspoon fresh dill, chopped
1-1/2 tablespoons fresh parsley, chopped
4 tablespoons red wine vinegar
4 tablespoons extra virgin olive oil
Sea salt and black pepper, to taste

PREPARATION
Deseed and slice the cucumbers and place them in a large bowl. Fold in diced tomatoes and onions. Sprinkle the fresh herbs, and season with salt and pepper. Add the vinegar and olive oil, and toss to mix.

Prep time 15 minutes. *Total time* 1-1/4 hours.

Serves 6

Notes

Early Spring Vegetables

This salad's colorful combination of carrots, red cabbage, spinach, and romaine represents early Spring's healthful bounty.

SHOPPING LIST
2 cups carrots, grated
1 cup red cabbage, shredded
1 cup turnip, grated
1 cup romaine, shredded
1 cup spinach leaves, torn
1/2 cup radishes, sliced
1 small red onion, sliced and separated into rings
Ground black pepper salt, to taste

PREPARATION
We recommend using a mandolin or benriner to shred the cabbage and slice the radishes and onions; the uniform cuts these tools help you produce allow the dressing to adequately penetrate each forkful. Place all the vegetables in a large bowl. Toss the vegetables in a lemon vinaigrette and season with salt and pepper. Serve the salad relatively soon after dressing it to avoid wilted spinach and soggy romaine.

Prep time 30 minutes

Serves 6

Notes

Winter Wheat Berry Salad
with Orange, Cauliflower, and Dried Fruit

This colorful winter salad highlights fragrant citrus, tender cauliflower, and summer's preserved fruits. The whole grain backdrop of wheat berry and rice will fill you up with lean protein and carbohydrate. While we enjoy the sturdy texture of wheat berries set against the softer rice grain, other ingredients in the salad can be paired with virtually any grain to yield a nourishing lunch or side dish. Try millet, black lentils, wild rice, or barley as a substitute for the wheat berries.

SHOPPING LIST
3 cups cooked wheat berries
3 cups cooked brown rice
2 teaspoons grated orange peel
1/4 cup plus 2 tablespoons sherry vinegar
1/4 cup plus 2 tablespoons extra virgin olive oil
2 naval oranges, segmented and zested
1 small head cauliflower, cut into florets
1 cup purple cabbage, shredded
3/4 cup dried apricots, chopped
1/4 cup pistachios, roasted and chopped
1/4 cup raisins
1/4 cup dried cranberries
Salt and pepper, to taste

Garnish
1/4 cup parsley, chopped

PREPARATION
Mix the wheat berries and rice in a large bowl. In a jar with tight fitting lid, combine the orange zest and segments, sherry vinegar, salt, and oil; shake to mix and pour the vinaigrette over the wheat berry mixture. Steam the cauliflower over boiling

water for 3–6 minutes. Mix the cauliflower, apricots, pistachios, cranberries, and raisins into the grains. Add salt and pepper to taste, garnish with parsley, and serve.

Prep time 2-1/4 hours

Serves 10

Notes

Pasta Primavera With Green Vegetables and Herbs

Aromatic herbs and spring vegetables make pasta primavera enticing as the sunlight hours extend into the evening and everything turns green. You can serve this dish either hot or cold, just be sure to mix the ingredients completely again before serving the pasta cold.

SHOPPING LIST
2 pounds dried penne
4 garlic cloves, minced
1 cup carrots, diced
1 cup celery, diced
1 cup onion, diced
1 cup broccoli, chopped fine
1 cup peas
1 cup fennel bulb, chopped fine
1 teaspoon coriander seeds, toasted and ground
1 teaspoon fennel seeds, toasted and ground
1-2 tablespoons olive oil
Salt and black pepper, to taste
Lemon vinaigrette
Garnish
1/4 cup fresh parsley minced
1/4 cup fresh basil minced
1/4 cup black olives, sliced

PREPARATION
Bring 3 quarts of water to a boil. Add the pasta, cook it until al dente, and then drain. Prepare the vinaigrette. Dice and chop your vegetables while you wait for the water to boil and the pasta to cook. In a large sauté pan, add a little oil and sweat the garlic, celery, onions, carrots, and spices until slightly soft and translucent. Add the broccoli and peas and cook until tender. When the pasta is *al dente*, drain it completely, place it

in the sauté pan, and stir until the vegetables coat the pasta. Add the vinaigrette and mix it into the pasta. Stir in sliced black olives and fresh herbs. You can serve Pasta Primavera hot or cold.

Prep time 1 hour

Serves 15

Notes:

Udon with Spiced Shrimp and Ginger

If you can find a decent quality product at your local store, purchase fresh shrimp. If you cannot find fresh shrimp, take a close look at the frozen product and its region of origin before purchasing; shrimp raised in farms outside the United States do not undergo the same sanitation and feeding requirements we expect from our seafood. Recently, chloramphenicol, an antibiotic banned in shrimp feed in our country, has been found in imported shrimp. Crawfish makes an excellent substitute for the shrimp in this recipe.

SHOPPING LIST
Dressing
2 garlic cloves, minced
4 tablespoons rice vinegar
1/4 cup soy sauce
1 teaspoon Dijon mustard
2 teaspoons fresh ginger, grated
1/4 teaspoon red pepper flakes
1/4 cup olive oil
Salt and ground pepper, to taste

Main Ingredients
1/2 pound Udon noodles
1 pound cooked shrimp (small size)
3 cucumbers, seeded and diced
2 scallions, white part only, sliced (reserve tops for garnish)
1 cup sliced snow pea pods, sliced in thirds
6 leaves red cabbage
Salt, to taste

Garnish
2 tablespoons toasted sesame seeds
Scallion tops, sliced

PREPARATION

In a small stainless steel bowl, assemble all the dressing ingredients except the oil. Then gradually whisk in the oil until blended. Bring a large pot of water to boil. Add the noodles to the boiling water, and cook until al dente. Rinse the noodles under cold water and drain. Place the noodles in a large bowl. Add the shrimp, cucumbers, scallions, snow peas, and dressing. Toss the ingredients until the noodles shine with the dressing and cling to the vegetables. Line a salad bowl with cabbage leaves. Lift the noodles and shrimp into the bowl; garnish with the sesame seeds and scallion tops.

Prep time 30 minutes.

Serves 6 to 8

Notes

Mid-Summer Vegetable Salad

You can keep the delicate flavors of green beans and summer squash intact by briefly cooking the vegetables in salted water and immediately cooling them in a salted ice bath. With a bright lemon vinaigrette, this salad allows each summer vegetable to retain its unique flavor and texture.

SHOPPING LIST
1 cup fresh corn (if you can't find fresh, canned will do)
1 cup green beans, cut in half
1 cup yellow squash, sliced into disks
1 cup red bell pepper, thinly sliced
1/2 cup onion, thinly sliced
1 cup lemon vinaigrette
Salt and ground black pepper, to taste

PREPARATION
Bring a small pot of water to boil and season the water with salt. Working in separate batches, blanch (submerge) your squash and green beans in the boiling water until they are cooked, but still have a bite and crunch. Pull the vegetables from the water with a slotted spoon or a spider, and plunge them into an ice water bath until cool. Drain the squash and green beans and place them in a large bowl—use a clean paper towel to make sure no water still clings to the vegetables. Sauté the corn in a little olive oil and salt, and once kernels cool, place them in the bowl with the remaining vegetables. Add the vinaigrette, and season and taste with salt and black pepper. Chill for one hour.

Prep time 30 minutes. *Total time* 1-1/2 hours.

Serves 4

Soups, Chilis, & Stews

Summer Vegetable Soup With Fresh Basil and Garlic

This straightforward vegetable soup captures summer's energy with a blast of fresh basil and garlic to garnish. While it is great any time you have fresh vegetables, you must try this soup when your herb garden has a bumper crop of fresh basil.

SHOPPING LIST
Main ingredients
1-1/2 tablespoons extra virgin olive oil
1/2 cup brown rice
1/2 pound fresh vegetables, such as green beans, trimmed
    and cut in half; zucchini, cut into thin sticks; peas, hulled
3-4 fresh carrots, medium diced
4 new potatoes, medium diced
Hot water to cover, about 2 quarts
Salt and ground pepper, to taste

Pistou
4-5 cloves garlic minced
1 cup basil leaves
1 teaspoon pine nuts (pignoli)
1-2 tablespoons extra virgin olive oil
1 lemon, zested

PREPARATION
In a stockpot add the oil, rice, and onions, and cook the mixture on a low flame until the onions soften. Add the salt and pepper and pour enough hot water over the vegetables to submerge them in the liquid. Bring the soup to a boil, reduce to a simmer, cover, add the potatoes, and cook for 5-10 minutes.

   Meanwhile, in a blender or food processor, blend together all the ingredients for the pistou until it forms a paste. You may need to add more oil. If you do, add 1/2 teaspoon and blend again. Set pistou aside.

Taste the rice; you should find a slight give against your tooth, but still some hard starchy resistance. Add the carrots, cook the mixture for 5 minutes, and then add the other vegetables; let the soup simmer until the vegetables are cooked but still retain a little snap. Remove from the heat. Ladle the soup into bowls, stir the pistou into each serving, and serve.

Prep time 1 hour.

Serves 4.

Notes

Summer Minestrone with Zucchini and Acni de Pepi

Sometimes the classic dishes don't need to be dressed up or distorted. Minestrone uses fresh seasonal vegetables, which allow you to eat until you can't eat any more without sacrificing health.

SHOPPING LIST

2 quarts vegetable stock	2 cloves garlic, minced
2 cups tomatoes, chopped	1 cup potatoes, diced
1 cup carrots, sliced	1 cup parsley, chopped
1 cup celery, sliced	2 cups zucchini, sliced
1 cup onion, diced	1-1/2 cups cooked red kidney
beans	
3 tablespoons red wine	1/4 cup cooked acni de pepe

Salt and ground pepper, to taste

Garnish
1 tablespoon parsley
1 tablespoon extra virgin olive oil
Shaved parmesan cheese, to taste

PREPARATION
Place the stock, tomatoes, carrots, celery, onion, wine, oregano, garlic, salt, and pepper in an 8-quart pot. Bring these ingredients to a boil, reduce to a simmer, and cook uncovered for about 40 minutes. Add the potatoes. Cook for about 20 minutes or until potatoes are tender. Add the zucchini and beans and cook for another 5-10 minutes, or until the zucchini is cooked, but not mushy. Cook the pasta separately, drain, toss in a little olive oil, and let it cool by spreading flat on a plate. Add the pasta to each serving bowl to avoid overcooking it. Finish the minestrone with parsley, extra virgin olive oil, and a few shards of Parmesan cheese.

Prep time 1-1/2 hours.

Serves 8

Notes

Cucumber Soup With Fresh Dill and Yogurt

Rose's favorite soup for festive occasions, this soup never fails to get rave reviews. If you plan to freeze portions of the soup, eliminate the dill, nonfat yogurt, vinegar, and cream of wheat; add these ingredients before you serve the soup to preserve the fresh taste.

SHOPPING LIST
16 medium-sized cucumbers, cut in half, seeded, and then cut into 1-inch chunks
6 leeks, cut in half and sliced (be sure to submerge in cold water to rinse)
8 shallots, small diced
1 large onion, medium diced
8 garlic cloves, minced
1 quart chicken or vegetable stock
1/4 cup fresh dill, chopped
1/2 cup nonfat yogurt
2 tablespoons champagne vinegar
2 tablespoons cream of wheat
Salt, to taste

PREPARATION
Peel and cut the cucumbers, thoroughly wash and slice the leeks, peel and crush the garlic and shallots. Place the leeks, shallots, garlic, and salt in a large stockpot and sauté until the vegetables are translucent and soft. Add the stock, bring it to a boil, and then add the cucumbers, and, if necessary, cream of wheat to thicken the soup. Cook for 5-8 minutes, or until the mixture boils again and the cucumbers soften. Pass the soup through a food mill or food processor. Season to taste with salt and vinegar. Add the fresh dill and yogurt before serving. Cucumber soup can be served cold or hot.

Prep time 1-1/2 hours.

Serves 8.

Notes

Smooth Black Bean Soup with Lime

Black beans contain the antioxidant anthocyanin, a generous amount of fiber, and when pureed offer a smoothness that rivals cream or butter-based soups. This recipe calls for dry black beans, so plan to soak the beans overnight before making the soup. If you don't have time for the overnight soak, canned black beans offer a quick alternative, but be sure to drain the beans through a colander and rinse them in running water before adding them to the soup. If you used canned beans, adjust the recipe by adding a quart of vegetable stock in place of the nutrient-rich bean water.

SHOPPING LIST
1 cup dry black beans
6 cups water or vegetable stock
1 onion, chopped
2 teaspoons olive oil
2 stalks celery, diced
2 carrots, diced
1 large potato, diced
4 large garlic cloves, minced
4 large shallots, minced
1 teaspoon fresh oregano
1/2 teaspoon black pepper
2 tablespoons lime juice
1 tablespoon lime zest
1 bay leaf
Salt to taste

Garnish
¼ cup nonfat yogurt
2 tablespoons chives, sliced

PREPARATION

Rinse and soak beans in a quart and a half of water overnight. Pour off the water and put the beans in a pot with 6 cups of water or stock and the bay leaf. Simmer the beans until tender, approximately one and a-half-hours. Cook the onion in olive oil until soft. Add diced celery, carrot, potato, and constantly stir the mixture so it cooks evenly. Add the vegetables to the cooked beans, along with the garlic, shallots, oregano, and black pepper. Simmer for one hour. Add the lime zest. Puree the soup in a food mill, processor, or blender until smooth. Return the soup to the pot and stir in the lime juice and salt. Reheat if necessary before serving. Garnish with a drizzle of yogurt and sliced chives.

Prep time 3 hours.

Serves 8.

Notes

Cabbage and Chickpea Minestra

Chunky vegetable soups will heal you and fill you up. This version combines the powerful antioxidant potential of tomatoes and cabbage. High in fiber, chickpeas (also known as garbanzo, or ceci beans) provide smooth substantial texture that will satiate your hunger.

SHOPPING LIST
2 teaspoons olive oil
1 large onion, chopped
3 garlic cloves, minced
1 cup tomatoes, chopped
2 cups cabbage, sliced
1 large potato, diced
4 cups water or vegetable stock
2 cups cooked chickpeas
1 teaspoon caraway, toasted and ground
1 teaspoon fennel, toasted and ground
Ground black pepper and salt, to taste

PREPARATION
In a large pot, sauté the onions and garlic in olive oil until they are soft and translucent. Add the tomatoes, potatoes, spices, and liquid. Once the soup comes to a simmer, add the beans and cabbage. Simmer until the vegetables are tender, approximately 5-8 minutes. Blend 3 cups of the soup until smooth. Return the pureed cups to the pot, stir to mix, and add salt and pepper to taste.

Prep time 45 minutes.

Serves 6.

Notes

Pumpkin Spice Soup

Ideally, you should try to find fresh pumpkin for this recipe, quarter and deseed the pumpkin, and roast it in the oven until cooked through. If you can't find fresh edible pumpkin, the following recipe uses canned pumpkin to create a surprisingly quick and delicious soup.

SHOPPING LIST
1 tablespoon olive oil
4 garlic cloves, minced
1 large onion, diced
1/8 teaspoon cayenne
1/2 teaspoon cumin
1/2 teaspoon ginger
1/2 teaspoon turmeric
2 cups water or vegetable stock
1 15-ounce can pumpkin
1-2 tablespoons honey
2 cups skim milk (or unsweetened soymilk)
1 tablespoon lemon juice
Salt, to taste

Garnish
5 fresh sage leaves, lightly toasted and chopped

PREPARATION
Heat the oil in a large pot, add the onion and garlic, and cook over low heat until the onion is soft. Add the turmeric, cayenne, cumin, ginger, and salt. Stir constantly. Add the water or vegetable stock, pumpkin, honey, and lemon juice. Simmer for 15 minutes.

Bring the soup to a simmer, check for seasoning, and remove from the stove. Puree the soup in a food processor, blender, or food mill until smooth. Stir in skim or unsweetened soymilk. Return the mixture to the pot and heat over medium heat until hot, but not boiling. Spoon into soup bowls and sprinkle with toasted sage before serving.

Prep time 1 hour.

Serves 6.

Notes

Mickey's Chicken Soup

Some of Rose and Sara's fondest memories are entering their mother's house welcomed by the aromas of this simple soup. By cooking the whole chicken in the soup's liquid, the flavors of the bird release into the stock and infuse it with wholesome richness.

SHOPPING LIST
1 soup chicken, cut into parts and skinned
2 large onions, diced
3 celery stalks with leaves, diced
4 large carrots, diced
1 small tomato, diced
5 garlic cloves, minced
2 teaspoons coriander
1/2 teaspoon fresh black pepper
1/2 teaspoon fresh basil
1/2 teaspoon fresh oregano
1/2 teaspoon fresh parsley
5 quarts water
1 cup rice or acini de pepe
Salt, to taste

PREPARATION
Wash the chicken, and place it in a large stockpot with the water, salt, and diced vegetables. Bring the stock to a boil, reduce the heat, and simmer for one hour. Remove the chicken from the broth. Cool, debone, dice the chicken, and then return it to the pot. Add the spices, bring the soup to a low boil, and add the rice or acine de pepe. Simmer the soup 10-15 minutes, or until the rice is cooked. Turn off the heat, add the fresh herbs, and serve.

Prep time 2-1/2 hours

Serves 10

Notes

Green Silk

Green vegetables such as broccoli and spinach contain high levels of lutein, a proven antioxidant. We know that a diet rich in these vegetables will help you fight cancer and live a strong life. The flavors and textures in this soup will leave you feeling as full as if you just ate a bacon-wrapped medallion of beef, but without the fat and fear that an unhealthy meal causes.

SHOPPING LIST
1 large onion, diced
2 celery stalks, diced
2 potatoes, diced
2 shallots, diced
1 cup split peas
6 cups water or vegetable stock
2 medium zucchini, diced
1 stalk broccoli, chopped
4 cups spinach, chopped
1 teaspoon fresh basil, chopped
1/2 teaspoon black pepper
1 tablespoon champagne vinegar
Salt to taste

PREPARATION
Sauté the onions and celery until translucent. Add the split peas in a large pot with the stock (or water), and bring to a boil. Reduce the heat and simmer for one hour. Add the potatoes. About 10 to 15 minutes later, when your potatoes are almost cooked through, add the zucchini, broccoli, spices, and simmer for 5-10 minutes. Take the soup off the heat. Add the spinach to the soup as you puree it in a food processor, blender, or food mill until smooth. Return the pureed soup to the pot; adjust the seasoning, add the champagne vinegar, and reheat to serve, if necessary. If you plan on making this soup several hours before

serving it, hold off on adding the champagne vinegar until right before serving—the acid might cause the vibrant green color to darken.

Prep time 1-3/4 hours

Serves 10.

Notes

Golden Beet and Potato Soup

Beets contain pigments called betalains that an act as antioxidants and have anticancer activity in the laboratory. These pigments can be yellow, orange, red, or purple red. This soup uses garden-fresh beets, potatoes, and dill to create a light first course or lunch.

SHOPPING LIST
8 medium gold beets, peeled and diced
4 large Yukon gold potatoes, diced
1 medium yellow onion, diced
6 cups water or vegetable stock
1/2 teaspoon black pepper
2 garlic cloves, minced
1 teaspoon olive oil
1/2 tablespoon fresh dill, chopped
Salt, to taste

PREPARATION
Crush the garlic into the olive oil and let the oil marinate while you start the soup. Put the vegetables in a large pot, add the vegetable stock, salt, and pepper, and bring the liquid to a boil. Reduce the heat and simmer the soup until the vegetables are tender and falling apart. Use a masher to crush the beets and potatoes until half of the soup is mashed. Add the minced garlic oil, and stir. Garnish each bowl with a pinch of fresh dill.

Prep time 45 minutes.

Serves 6.

Notes

Butternut Squash, Carrot, and Ginger Soup

The aromas of ginger, cinnamon, cumin, turmeric, and garlic simmering in olive oil will entice even the most reluctant vegetable eaters. This recipe uses apple cider vinegar to balance the sweetness of carrot and squash. Ginger and cinnamon, powerful antioxidants, combine with the carotenoids in squash to support your health.

SHOPPING LIST
1 tablespoon olive oil
3-4 garlic cloves, minced
2 shallots, diced
2 tablespoons ginger, shredded
1/8 teaspoon turmeric
1/8 teaspoon cumin
1/8 teaspoon cinnamon
8 carrots, sliced
3 cups butternut squash, cubed
5 cups water
1/2 cup apple cider

Garnish
1/8 teaspoon cinnamon
1 strip of crystallized ginger, shaved or thinly sliced

PREPARATION
In a large pot, sauté the garlic and shallots in olive oil until translucent. Add the shredded ginger and spices, and cook for three minutes. Stir in the carrots and squash. Cook for 5 minutes. Add the water and cider. Cover the pot and simmer for 45 minutes. Be sure to stir the pot occasionally to avoid scorching on the bottom. Turn off the heat and puree the soup in a food processor, food mill, or blender until smooth. Return

the soup to the pot and reheat if necessary. Garnish with a dash of cinnamon and a thin shave of crystallized ginger.

Prep time 1 hour.

Serves 6.

Notes

Yellow and Green Split Pea Soup

If you are busy this soup can be cooked in a crock-pot as you run errands. While traditional split pea soups get their richness from smoked ham hocks, we offer a healthy alternative with fragrant vegetables and spices.

SHOPPING LIST
1 cup green split peas
1 cup yellow split peas
6 cups water, vegetable or chicken broth
1 large onion, chopped
1 large leek, cut in half and sliced
3 garlic cloves, minced
2 shallots, chopped
2 large carrots, diced
2 celery stalks, diced
1 large potato, diced
1/8 teaspoon ground cloves
1/4 teaspoon ground cumin
Salt and black pepper, to taste

PREPARATION
Peel and mince, chop, slice, and dice vegetables. Be sure to clean the sliced leeks by submerging them in cold water and lifting them out with a slotted spoon. Rinse the peas and put them into a large stockpot with all the ingredients. Bring to a simmer, cover loosely, and cook until the peas are tender (approximately one hour). Or put the ingredients in a crock-pot and let them slowly cook. Blend one half of the soup and return it to the pot. Check for seasoning and serve the soup with a drizzle of extra virgin olive oil.

Prep time 1-1/4 hours.

Serves 8.

Notes

Butternut Squash Soup

Last year we planted our own butternut squash at Buck Mountain Farms, and we had many pounds of bright orange sweetness to experiment with. This soup takes a different approach to butternut squash soup than our earlier recipe, and seeks to highlight the squash's bright flavor with the addition of warm spices. Butternut squash and pumpkin contain high levels of carotinoids, which offer multiple health benefits.

SHOPPING LIST
4 pounds butternut squash
2-3 quarts vegetable stock
1/8 teaspoon cardamom
1 tablespoon brown sugar (optional)
1/8 teaspoon allspice
1/8 teaspoon cinnamon
1/8 teaspoon nutmeg
Salt, to taste

Garnish
24 sage leaves

PREPARATION
Preheat oven to 375°F. Cut the squash in half, clean it of seeds and pulp, and place it flesh side down on an oiled and salted sheet tray. Cook the squash until soft. Take the squash out of the oven, flip it over, and let it cool. Once cooled, scrape the squash flesh from the skin, add it to a large pot with 2-3 quarts of stock, and stir to mix the liquid and squash. Add the spices and salt and simmer for 1/2 hour.

Garnish with oven-crisped sage leaves.

Prep time 45 minutes. *Total time* 2 hours.

Serves 8.

Notes

Potato Soup with Green Peppers and Chili

A warm and slightly spicy potato soup offers a delightful way of staying comfortable as the cold weather brings rain, snow, and wind. Since the spicy heat of chilies will vary depending on the variety available at the local market, you will want to adjust the amount you put into the soup to your taste.

SHOPPING LIST
3-4 large Yukon Gold potatoes, diced
4 cups water
1 tablespoon olive oil
1 large onion, diced
3 garlic cloves, minced
1 large green bell pepper, diced
1 teaspoon cumin
1/2 teaspoon coriander
1 teaspoon fresh basil, chopped
1/2 teaspoon black pepper
2 poblano peppers, diced (or two ancho peppers, ground)
2 cups skim milk (or unsweetened soymilk)
2 scallions, sliced thin
1/4 nonfat yogurt, whisked to thin
Salt to taste

PREPARATION
Starting with cold water, heat the diced potatoes in a covered pot until tender. Mash the potatoes in the cooking water and leave some chunks for contrasting texture. Set aside to cool. Heat the oil in a large pot and cook the onion until soft. Add the garlic, bell and poblano pepper, and spices. Cook the vegetables for 5 minutes, or until tender. Add the potatoes with the cooking liquid. Be sure to stir in the potato so that the bottom of the pot doesn't burn. Add the milk. Continually heat the soup until it gently simmers. Check the seasoning for

salt. Garnish with the chopped scallions and a drizzle of thinned yogurt in each bowl.

Prep time 45 minutes.

Serves 8.

Notes

Chocolate Chili

This recipe borrows chocolate from Mexican mole sauces to accelerate the antioxidant power of a robust chili. Chocolate chili is a favorite dish at our family farm because of its simplicity and taste. This dish freezes well. We make a large batch and freeze meal-sized portions that we use for lunches. The chili powder lends heat to this dish. You can control the heat by selecting mild, medium, or hot chili powder.

SHOPPING LIST
1 large onion, chopped
1 large green bell pepper, seeded and chopped
1tablespoon olive oil
1 tablespoon whole mustard seed
1 2-ounce square of dark chocolate (check for no milk fat)
1/2 teaspoon cinnamon
2 tablespoons chili powder
1 teaspoon cumin seeds, ground
1 16-ounce can crushed tomatoes
2 16 ounce cans pinto or red beans, drained and rinsed
2 cups vegetable broth
1 6-ounce can tomato paste
Salt and pepper, to taste

Garnish
1/4 cup nonfat sour cream
1/4 cup scallions, sliced thin

PREPARATION
In a large saucepan, sauté the onion and green pepper in the olive oil until the vegetables begin to caramelize. Add the mustard seed and cook for 2 minutes. Add the chili powder, cumin seed, chocolate, cinnamon, tomatoes, beans, broth, salt, pepper, and tomato paste. While continually stirring, simmer the

chili for about 35 minutes until the mixture thickens. Garnish the chili with nonfat sour cream and scallions.

Prep time 1-1/4 hours.

Serves 6.

Notes

Summer Vegetable Chili

Black soybeans get their stark color from the antioxidant anthocyanin. This chili combines black soybeans with pinto and white beans for a visually stunning vegetable chili. Try this recipe in midsummer, when fresh local zucchini, yellow squash, and corn fill the markets.

SHOPPING LIST
1/2 cup vegetable stock
1/2 cup onion, chopped
1/2 cup green bell pepper, small diced
1/2 cup corn
2 pounds of skinned and seeded tomatoes,
   or 1 28-ounce can of stewed tomatoes
1 cup black soybeans, cooked
1 cup pinto beans, cooked
1 cup white beans, cooked
1 cup green chilies, chopped
1/2 pound firm tofu drained, diced
1/2 cup zucchini, large diced
1/2 cup yellow straight-necked squash, large diced
1 tablespoon chili powder
1/8 teaspoon cayenne powder
Salt and pepper, to taste

Garnish
1/4 cup nonfat sour cream
1/4 cup scallions

PREPARATION
Put the stock, onion, and green pepper in a large stockpot. Bring the liquid to a boil and stir in the remaining ingredients. Season to taste with salt and pepper. Reduce the mixture to a simmer and cook uncovered for about 20 minutes. Add the

zucchini, squash, and tofu, and simmer for another 15 minutes. Serve in the chili in soup bowls and garnish with nonfat sour cream and scallions. Alternatively, you can serve the chili over brown rice for a filling meal.

Prep time 1 hour.

Serves 8.

Notes

Barley and Lentil Stew With Fresh Herbs

Traditionally paired with beef and beef stock, barley and lentils stand up on their own in this vegetable-based spiced stew.

SHOPPING LIST
1 cup green lentils
1/2 cup pearled barley
6 cups water or vegetable stock
1 medium onion, diced
4 garlic cloves, minced
2 celery stalks, diced
3 carrots, diced
1-2 tablespoons olive oil
1/2 teaspoon fresh oregano
1/2 teaspoon cumin
1/4 teaspoon coriander
1/2 teaspoon black pepper
Salt and pepper, to taste

Garnish
2 teaspoons Tabasco sauce
2 tablespoons parsley, chopped

PREPARATION
Sauté the onions, garlic, celery, and carrots in olive oil until translucent and tender. Add the spices, oregano, and salt—but not the Tabasco and parsley. Add the barley and stir until each grain is coated in oil. Add the stock, bring to a boil, and simmer for 30 minutes. Add the lentils and bring the liquid to a boil before reducing to a simmer and covering. Cook for 30 minutes, checking occasionally to see if the barley and lentils are cooked. Finish the stew by stirring in the Tabasco (you may want to add a few more drops, depending on the amount of spice you like.) Garnish each bowl with a pinch of fresh parsley.

Prep time 1-1/4 hours.

Serves 8.

Notes

Couscous and Chickpea Stew with Tomatoes and Peppers

This is a quintessential Mediterranean stew, full of flavor from the harmonious combination of spices and summer vegetables. While this recipe includes directions for roasting your own peppers, this can be time-consuming. You can purchase peppers already roasted in most large grocery stores and at some of the online sources we list elsewhere in this book.

SHOPPING LIST
1 large eggplant, sliced
1 pound small new potatoes, cut in half
2 cups vegetable broth
2 tablespoons balsamic vinegar
1 large onion, chopped
2 shallots, chopped
2 tablespoon ginger, grated
1 teaspoon cumin, ground
1 teaspoon coriander, ground
1/4 teaspoon cinnamon
1/2 teaspoon saffron
2 red bell peppers, roasted, peeled, and sliced
1 green bell pepper, roasted, peeled, and sliced
1 yellow bell pepper, roasted, peeled, and sliced
3 cups chickpeas, cooked
1-1/2 cups fresh Roma tomatoes, peeled, seeded, and chopped
1/2 cup raisins
1-1/2 cups couscous
Salt and pepper, to taste

Garnish
1/4 cup cucumber, deseeded, grated, and drained
1/4 cup fresh basil, minced

PREPARATION

Under a broiler roast the peppers until their skin chars; remove them from the broiler and place them in a stainless steel bowl. Tightly seal the bowl in plastic wrap. Set the peppers aside for 30-40 minutes, or until the skin easily pulls from the flesh. Peel the skin and scrape the seeds out of the peppers. Place salted eggplant slices on a baking sheet slathered with olive oil and bake them at 425°F until tender (do not let them get too soft). Remove the eggplant from the oven and cool. In the meantime, bring a large pot of water to a boil, add the potatoes, reduce and simmer. When tender, pull the potatoes from the water and set them to cool on a plate. In a large skillet, simmer the broth and vinegar, and then add the shallots, ginger, onion, cumin, coriander, cinnamon, and saffron. Season to taste with salt and pepper. Simmer the vegetables and spices until the liquid almost evaporates. Stir in the peppers and chickpeas to mix thoroughly. Add the tomatoes and mix until the pan's liquid is reduced to a thick sauce. Stir in the raisins, eggplant, and potatoes. Reduce the heat to a simmer and cover. Cook for 10 minutes. Add two tablespoons of broth at a time to prevent scorching. In the meantime, prepare the couscous. In a medium saucepan bring 1-1/2 cups of water to a boil. Place the couscous in a large pot with a little salt and oil. Pour the boiling water over the couscous, cover and let stand for 20 minutes. Fluff the couscous with a fork and transfer it to a serving platter. Make a deep well in the center and place the fragrant stew in the well. Garnish with grated cucumber, fresh basil, and a drizzle of extra virgin olive oil.

Prep time 2 hours.

Serves 4.

Notes

Green Lentil, Barley, and White Bean Stew with Tomato and Herbs

If you can find French green lentils, we recommend using them; they hold their shape and unique texture longer than other lentils, which tend to get mushy if overcooked.

SHOPPING LIST
2 tablespoons olive oil
4 carrots, medium diced
2 leeks, medium
2 ribs of celery, medium diced
1 large onion, chopped
2 medium zucchini, medium diced
2-3 garlic cloves, minced
1 tablespoon fresh thyme leaves
1 cup French green lentils, rinsed
1/2 cup pearled barley, rinsed
1/2 cup cooked white beans
7 cups vegetable stock
2 cups tomatoes, peeled, chopped, and seeded
1/2 cup fresh basil, torn
1/2 cup parsley, chopped
Salt and pepper, to taste

PREPARATION
Place the olive oil in a large pot and add the carrots, leeks, celery, onion, and garlic. Season the vegetables to taste with ground pepper and salt, and cook them over low heat until they become translucent. Add the barley and stock. Bring the liquid to a boil, reduce to a simmer, and cook for 10 minutes; then add the lentils, and let the soup simmer for 30 minutes.

Add the tomatoes, zucchini, and cooked white beans and simmer for 10 more minutes, or until the lentils and barley are cooked through. Check for seasoning, and garnish with parsley and basil.

Prep time 1-1/4 hours.

Serves 6.

Notes

Ratatouille

In traditional versions of Ratatouille you cook each vegetable separately before mixing them together for a brief simmer. This allows each ingredient to retain its individual flavor. While nothing can compare with the original version's distinct flavor, we have adapted the recipe so it is quick and easy to follow after a long day of work. An antioxidant powerhouse packed with lycopene, you can serve ratatouille over pasta or generously spread it on grilled bread.

SHOPPING LIST
4 medium eggplants, medium diced
2 tablespoons extra virgin olive oil
4 onions, sliced
2 fennel bulbs, chopped
8 garlic cloves, minced
2 red bell peppers, roasted and sliced
12 ripe tomatoes, peeled, seeded, and chopped
2 tablespoons parsley
1 tablespoon thyme
2 bay leaves
1 teaspoon rosemary
2 zucchini, medium diced
Salt and pepper, to taste

PREPARATION
On a well-oiled sheet tray, place eggplant in a single layer and bake at 425°F, until browned on the top. Flip the eggplant dices over and remove them from oven to cool. Sauté the onions, fennel, and garlic in a large well-oiled skillet. Stir in the bell peppers, tomatoes, bay leaves, thyme, and rosemary. Season the vegetables to taste with salt and pepper. Simmer the mixture until it becomes thick and saucy, about 25 minutes. Stir in the zucchini and cook it until tender. Meanwhile, mix in the roasted

eggplant. Finish the ratatouille with a drizzle of extra-virgin olive oil and parsley.

Prep time 1-1/4 hours.

Serves 8.

Notes

Mushroom, Chard, and Barley Stew

Maitake mushrooms might be hard to locate at some markets, but if you can find them they will add a complexity of flavor hard to find in other mushrooms. Dried shiitake mushrooms are now widely available in most stores, so if you cannot find maitake or oyster mushrooms, they make a great substitute.

SHOPPING LIST
3 large golden potatoes, diced
1 cup dried mushrooms (shiitake, maitake, or oyster)
1/2 cup pearled barley
1/4 pound red chard, chopped
4 quarts water
1 teaspoon hot Hungarian paprika
1/2 teaspoon hot curry powder
1/2 teaspoon ground coriander
1/2 teaspoon ginger
1/2 teaspoon turmeric
1/2 teaspoon marjoram (fresh or dried)
1 teaspoon fresh rosemary
1/2 teaspoon fresh thyme, chopped
1/5 cup soy sauce
3-4 cloves garlic, minced
Salt and pepper, to taste

Garnish
1/2 teaspoon fresh dill, chopped
1 tablespoon fresh basil, sliced thin or torn

PREPARATION
In a stockpot bring the water and mushrooms to a boil and add the barley. Reduce the heat to a simmer, add the spices and herbs (except the basil and dill), and cook for 45 minutes. Add the diced potatoes and cook the stew until the barley and

potatoes are tender. Five minutes before serving add the chard. Finish the stew with torn fresh basil, chopped dill, and a drizzle of extra-virgin olive oil.

Prep time: 1 hour.

Serves 4-6.

Notes

Green Olive, White Bean, and Potato Stew

This dish is a nutritional powerhouse. White beans provide healthy protein along with soluble fiber. The green olives are rich in oleuropein. This compound and its metabolite hydroxytyrosol have powerful antioxidant activity that preserves the oil of the olive and helps account for its multiple health benefits. Delicious variations on this dish can be prepared by adding various greens like spinach, chard, escarole or kale.

SHOPPING LIST
6 medium new potatoes, medium diced
1 tablespoon extra virgin olive oil
2 large onions, chopped
4 garlic cloves, minced
1 tablespoon oregano
2 tablespoons dry white wine
2 cups tomatoes, peeled, seeded, and chopped
4 cups white beans, cooked
8 pitted black olives, quartered
4 green olives, sliced
Salt and ground pepper, to taste

Garnish
2 tablespoons fresh basil, torn

PREPARATION
Starting with cold water, in a large stockpot gently simmer the potatoes until just cooked through, about 12 minutes. Lift the potatoes out of the water and cool. Heat olive oil in a large skillet and sauté the onions, garlic, and oregano until tender. Add the wine, stir, and cook to reduce. Stir in the tomatoes, and cook until the mixture starts to thicken. Add the white beans and simmer for 10 minutes. Add the potatoes, cover the pot, and continue to simmer the mixture for 5 minutes.

The resulting sauce should be thick and coat the beans. Add the sliced olives. Adjust the seasoning with salt and pepper. Garnish with torn basil and a drizzle of extra virgin olive oil.

Prep time 35 minutes.

Serves 6.

Porcini Mushrooms and Lentils With Parsnips

While fresh porcinis remain difficult to locate in many regions of the United States, dried porcinis can be found in most supermarkets or ordered online. Dried porcinis have a flavor concentration and deep earthiness that cannot be matched; this rich flavor makes them a natural fit for stews.

SHOPPING LIST
4 ounces dried porcinis
2-1/2 large onions, chopped
1 cup French green lentils
1 bay leaf
2 tablespoons extra virgin olive oil
4 garlic cloves, minced
2 leeks, chopped
2 teaspoons cumin, ground
1/2 teaspoon coriander, ground
1/4 teaspoon cinnamon, ground
2 tablespoons balsamic vinegar
2 parsnips, peeled and sliced
1 tablespoon whole wheat flour
1 pound firm tofu, diced

Garnish
1/4 cup parsley, chopped
1-2 teaspoons Tabasco sauce

PREPARATION
Re-hydrate the porcini mushrooms by simmering them in 3 cups of water for 30 minutes. Place the onions, leeks, garlic, and spices in a large saucepan with the olive oil, and sauté until tender. Chop the mushrooms and add them to the skillet. Sprinkle the flour over the mixture and stir to avoid clumping. Add the lentils, bay leaf, 2 cups of vegetable stock and the

remaining porcini liquid. Bring the lentil mixture to a boil, cover, and simmer for 30 minutes. Add the parsnips and simmer for 10 minutes. Add the diced tofu and cook for 5 minutes. Stir in the vinegar. Check the stew for appropriate doneness and seasoning. Garnish each bowl with fresh chopped parsley and a drop or two of Tabasco sauce.

Prep time 1 3/4 Hours.

Serves 6.

Notes

Entrees

Eggplant Casserole with Fresh Tomato and Black Olives

You can make an impressive list of various dishes with eggplants, fresh tomatoes, and olives. From antipasto, pasta sauces, and bruschetta toppings to tians and bread puddings, these three ingredients simply work together to create a sublime flavor balance. The following casserole adds egg whites and nonfat cheese to increase the overall protein content of the dish.

SHOPPING LIST
1 eggplant, unpeeled and sliced 1/3" thick
2 large ripe tomatoes, sliced thin
3 large hardboiled egg whites, sliced
1/2 cup nonfat mozzarella, shredded
1 cup fresh breadcrumbs
1/2 cup grated nonfat Pecorino Romano
3 garlic cloves, minced
3 tablespoons fresh basil, minced
3 tablespoons fresh parsley, minced
1 teaspoon oregano
1/3 cup black olives, sliced
2 tablespoons extra virgin olive oil

PREPARATION
Heat an oven to 425°F. Spread the eggplant slices in a single layer on a well-oiled baking sheet and cook them until tender. Oil an 8-inch baking dish. Remove the eggplant from the oven and transfer the slices to the baking dish, covering the bottom of the dish. Next, layer the tomatoes slices, sprinkle the olives, and distribute the cheese and eggs on top. In a food processor or blender, combine the breadcrumbs, Pecorino cheese, garlic, basil, oregano, and parsley. Sprinkle the mixture evenly over the casserole, and drizzle the top with olive oil. Cover the dish

with foil and bake for 15 minutes. Remove the foil and continue baking until the cheese melts and caramelizes, usually about ten minutes. Let the casserole set for ten minutes before serving. This dish works well made a day in advance and refrigerated.

Prep time 2-1/2 hours.

Serves 4.

Notes

Cauliflower Tofu Stir-fry with Thai Basil

Tofu takes on a savory sauce of tamari, ginger, garlic, and apple cider vinegar in this vibrant stir-fry. We've included kale and cauliflower to increase the antioxidant content of the recipe.

SHOPPING LIST

Marinade
2 tablespoons tamari soy sauce
1 tablespoon malt vinegar
2 teaspoons apple cider vinegar
3 garlic cloves, peeled and minced
1 tablespoon ginger, grated
1 tablespoon olive oil

Stir-fry
1 tablespoon olive oil
1 large onion, chopped
2 large garlic cloves, chopped
1 pound firm tofu, drained, cut into 1" cubes, and marinated
3 cups tightly packed chopped kale leaves
1-1/2 tablespoons mild curry powder
1/8 red pepper flakes
1-1/2 cups vegetable stock
1 large head of cauliflower, cut into florets
1 large red bell pepper, seeded and diced
1 teaspoon tamari soy sauce
1/4 cup Thai basil, torn

PREPARATION
Assemble the marinade and toss the tofu in the mixture. Marinade the tofu for 25 minutes in the refrigerator before cooking.

In a large skillet or wok, heat the oil and add the onion, garlic, and tofu. Stir-fry the mixture until the tofu begins to caramelize. Stir in the kale and sprinkle in the red pepper flakes and curry powder. Add 1/4 cup of the stock, cover, and simmer the mixture for 2 minutes. Then add the cauliflower, red pepper, and a teaspoon of tamari. Add 1/2 cup of the stock, cover, and continue to simmer, stirring every minute or so until the kale becomes tender and the cauliflower just cooked through, about 5 minutes. Add more stock as needed to prevent burning. Stir in the Thai basil. You can serve this stir-fry over rice, bulgur wheat, or couscous.

Prep time 45 minutes.

Serves 6.

Notes

Jaipur Chicken with Rice

Most Jaipur chicken recipes call for cream and coconut milk, but we've adapted the traditional recipe so you can enjoy it without the worry that dairy fat and products high in cholesterol bring. Besides the intensity of flavor and rich aromatics, another benefit of eating this dish is its use of turmeric. Turmeric contains curcumin, a powerful antioxidant, anti-inflammatory, and anticancer agent.

SHOPPING LIST
2 cups long grain brown basmati rice
1-2 tablespoons olive oil
2-1/2 –3 pounds skinned and de-boned chicken thighs
1 large onion, chopped
4 large garlic cloves, minced
1 tablespoon turmeric
1/4 teaspoon ground cumin
2 teaspoons fennel seeds
1/4 teaspoon cayenne pepper
1/2 teaspoon freshly ground black pepper
1/2 teaspoon paprika
1/2 cup vegetable stock
1 teaspoon lime zest
2 tablespoons lime juice
Salt and pepper, to taste

Garnish
1/4 cup fresh parsley, chopped

PREPARATION
Begin by fully cooking the rice in a pot of seasoned water. While the rice cooks, heat the olive oil in a large heavy skillet over medium heat. Season and lightly brown the chicken, adding a few pieces at a time until each piece slightly colors. (Do not

create a hard or dark crust on the chicken as this may cause carcinogens to develop on the meat's surface). Transfer all of the chicken to a plate. Blend all of the spices and garlic with the chicken stock and lime juice until smooth. In the skillet add the onion and sauté it, scraping the bottom and sides of the pan. Stir in the blended spice and garlic liquid. Add the lime zest to the pan. Return the chicken to the pan. Bring the mixture to a boil and then reduce it to a simmer. Cover. Occasionally baste the chicken until it is cooked through. Before serving, arrange the rice around the edges of a serving platter. Spoon the chicken mixture into the center. Garnish with fresh parsley.

Prep time 1-1/2 hours.

Serves 4.

Notes

Edamame and Quinoa with Pistachio

Quinoa has more quality protein than any other grain. The ancient Incans used quinoa to help power their long distance runners over the Andes Mountains. Edamame pairs naturally with this super-grain, and we've added a kick of red pepper and fresh herbs to brighten the dish.

SHOPPING LIST
1 large onion, chopped coarsely
4 garlic cloves, minced
1 tablespoon olive oil
2 cups vegetable stock
1-1/2 cups uncooked quinoa, rinsed
1-3/4 cups edamame (fresh or frozen, out of the pod)
1 teaspoon oregano, chopped
1 teaspoon red pepper flakes
Salt and black pepper, to taste

Garnish
2 tablespoons pistachios, roasted and chopped
2 tablespoons parsley, chopped
1 tablespoon bell pepper, diced finely

PREPARATION
In a stockpot, sauté the onion and garlic in olive oil until tender. Pour in the vegetable stock, quinoa, oregano, red pepper flakes, salt, and black pepper. Bring the mixture to a boil and then lower the heat and cover the pot. After the mixture has cooked for fifteen minutes, add the edamame. Simmer the mixture for 5 minutes, or until all liquid has been absorbed. Garnish with chopped pistachios, red pepper, and parsley.

Prep time 1/2 hour.

Serves 6.

Notes

Chicken Sausage with Tomatoes, Spinach, and Chickpeas

The following recipe packs an antioxidant power punch with spinach, chickpeas, and tomatoes. Spinach contains high levels of the antioxidant lutein; cooked tomatoes contain the antioxidant lycopene, and chickpeas provide fiber to help you feel full and satisfied. While the dish stands on its own, you can try it over pasta or rice for a more substantial meal.

SHOPPING LIST
3-4 uncured organic chicken sausages, sliced
4 garlic cloves, minced
1 tablespoon olive oil
3 cups chickpeas, cooked
1 large red onion, chopped
1 28-ounce can or jar of crushed tomatoes
1 cup Roma tomatoes, peeled, seeded, and chopped
1 tablespoon red pepper, crushed
1/8 teaspoon fennel seeds, toasted and ground
1 shallot, chopped
1 tablespoon oregano, chopped
1 tablespoon of lemon zest, chopped
Salt and black pepper, to taste

PREPARATION
In a large saucepan, sauté the onion and garlic in olive oil until translucent. Add the chickpeas, tomatoes, pepper flakes, ground fennel seed, shallot, lemon zest, salt, ground black pepper, and oregano. Bring the mixture to a simmer and cover for 15 minutes. Add the sliced chicken sausages, stir them into the mixture, and cook for 5-7 minutes or until heated through. (Many of these sausages are precooked, so you just need to heat them through—be careful not to overcook). Add the spinach and toss until just wilted.

Prep time 45 minutes.

Serves 8.

Notes

Spaghetti with Clams, Garlic, and Hot Pepper

Fresh clams and their brine become the sauce in this simple recipe. Make sure to wash your clams by running them under cold running water and scrub the shells if necessary. If you like eating clams in their shells and scooping up the liquid gold of the sauce, try arranging them so they are easily accessible on the top of the spaghetti or off to the side. Scallops, monkfish, or picked lobster and crab can be substituted for the clams in this recipe, but you will need to adjust the cooking time.

SHOPPING LIST
3 dozen Manila clams, washed and scrubbed
1-1/2 tablespoons olive oil
1 medium onion, finely chopped
3 large garlic cloves, minced
1/2 cup stock
1/2 cup dry white wine
1 bay leaf
1 pound whole wheat spaghetti
1/2 teaspoon ground or flaked red pepper

Garnish
1/4 cup chopped parsley
Extra virgin olive oil

PREPARATION
Heat a large saucepan and add olive oil, onions, and garlic. Sauté until translucent. Add the clams, stock, and wine and bring the liquid to a simmer. Briefly cover the pan until the clams begin to open. As each clam opens, pick it out with a pair of tongs and place it in a large bowl. If you desire shell-free clams in your pasta, remove the clam meat from the shells. Catch all the juices. Add the juices to the broth and boil until the liquid is reduced by about one third. In the meantime,

cook the pasta and drain it in a colander. Add the pasta to the broth, and let it sit for one minute to absorb the juices. Right before serving, add the clams and toss them until warmed through; or arrange the clamshells around the plate.

Finish with chopped parsley and a drizzle of extra virgin olive oil.

Prep time 45 minutes. *Total time* 1 hour.

Serves 4.

Notes

Spaghetti Marinara

A simple pasta sauce, marinara contains very high levels of lycopene to help you remain healthy and active. If you can find fresh tomatoes, try using them instead of the canned puree. Blanche the fresh tomatoes, briefly chill them in ice water, remove their skins and seeds, chop them up, and continue as directed in the following recipe.

SHOPPING LIST
1 pound spaghetti
2 tablespoons olive oil
1 quart tomato puree
5 garlic cloves, minced
1/4 teaspoon black pepper, ground
1 tablespoon fresh oregano, chopped
1 tablespoon fresh basil, torn
Salt to taste

PREPARATION
Slowly heat the olive oil in a saucepan, bloom the garlic in the oil, and add the oregano and tomato puree. Cook the sauce over low heat for 30 minutes or until thick enough to coat the noodles. Meanwhile, bring 3 quarts of salted water to a boil. Add the spaghetti, cook until al dente and then drain the noodles in a colander. Pour the sauce over the pasta, toss to thoroughly coat, and finish the spaghetti with torn basil.

To make this dish nutritionally more complete, add one or more of the following ingredients to the marinara sauce:

Meatless Meatballs (recipe on the next page)
1 cup cooked skinless chicken thighs, diced
1 cup lentils, cooked
1 cup tofu, diced

Prep time 45 minutes.

Serves 4.

Notes

Meatless Meatballs

Okay, so these aren't really meatballs, but we think you'll be fooled by the flavor. We have made this recipe for company and no one has ever guessed that they don't contain meat. They work great with the previously mentioned marinara sauce.

SHOPPING LIST
1 pound Silken tofu
1 cup breadcrumbs
1/2 cup onion, sautéed in olive oil until soft
1 tablespoon oregano, chopped
1 tablespoon basil, chopped
1 tablespoon fennel seed, ground
1/2 –1 teaspoon salt
1/2 teaspoon black pepper
5 garlic cloves, minced
1 teaspoon powdered garlic
½ cup egg whites

PREPARATION
In a large bowl mash the tofu and slowly add the egg whites and other ingredients. Mix very well. Mixture should be *slightly* dry. Form into 1" balls and brown in a skillet with a generous amount of olive oil. If you are worried about cooking with too much oil because of the extra calories, try baking the meatless meatballs in a 400°F, oven until browned. Add to marinara sauce and serve over pasta.

Prep time 20 minutes.

Serves 6.

Notes

Chicken Meatballs with Lemon and Sage

In this version, lemon zest brightens a traditional meatball recipe. Try these lemon and herb-scented meatballs with pesto, or mixed into sauteed spinach, garlic, and pasta. You can roll the mixture into small balls. After cooking squewer and then paint the meatballs with pesto for a scrumptous hor d'oeuvre.

SHOPPING LIST
1 tablespoon olive oil
3/4 cup onion, small diced
1/8 teaspoon crushed red pepper
1/2 cup white bread crumbs
1 tablespoon fresh sage, finely chopped
1-2 teaspoons salt
1/8 teaspoon black pepper, ground
1 meduim egg white
1 pound ground chicken

Preheat your oven to 400°F. Sautee onions in olive oil until translucent and allow to cool. Grind white bread in a food processor until small crumbs form and then soak in just enough unsweetened soy milk or milk to soften, about 5-10 minutes. After soaking the breadcrumbs, squeeze out the liquid and add the mush to the other ingredients in a large bowl. Make sure to evenly distribute the bread and egg whites along with the other ingredients. Place the mixture in a refrigerator for at least an hour before rolling out either small balls for hor d'oeuvres or larger balls for an entree. After rolling, you can either freeze the chicken meatballs for later use, or begin cooking them. Generously oil a large sheet tray or oven-safe glass dish. Place the meatballs on the tray with enough space so they will brown. Place the tray in the preheated oven. Check the doneness of the meatballs periodically; you want a cooked meatball, but keep in mind a dry meatball should be avoided. For smaller balls, 6-8 mintues should be fine. For larger balls, 8-15 mintues is likely. The balls should be slightly brown, set, and firm, but still juicy and moist.

Prep Time: 1-1/2 hours (This time includes an hour of rest in the refrigerator).

Serves: 3-4 entrée portions, or 5-7 hors d'oeuvres portions.

Notes

Veggie Burgers

The following recipe has been adapted from a series of recipes that appeared in *The Vegetarian Times*. The basic method will work with many ingredient variations. Once you make the 'dough' from overcooked pasta and beans, you can substitue rice, wheatberries, or barley for the quinoa, switch the cabbage and capers for olives and broccoli, or any vegetable similar in texture and flavor. Just make sure to shred or chop the vegetables so they match the size specifications outlined below.

SHOPPING LIST
4 ounces over-cooked pasta (farfalle, penne, or rigatoni)
1/4 cup quinoa
6 ounces vegetable or chicken broth
2 tablespoons olive oil for sauteing
3/4 cup yellow onion, small diced
4 garlic cloves, minced
1/2 cup carrot, small diced
1 15 ounce can garbonzo beans, rinsed, and drained of all liquid
1/3 cup red cabbage, finely shredded
2 tablespoons tomato sauce
2 teaspoons capers, finely chopped
1 teaspoon fresh oregano, finely chopped
2 teaspoons fresh parsley, finely chopped
1/4 teaspoon salt (more or less, to taste)
2 tablespoons pumpkin seeds, roasted and chopped

PREPARATION
Rinse the quinoa and place it in a pot with 6 ounces of vegetable or chicken broth. Cook the quinoa until done, but not blown out or waterlogged. Meanwhile, dice the carrot and onion and chop the garlic. Sautee these vegetables until translucent in one tablespoon of olive oil. Combine the

overcooked pasta, drained and rinsed garbanzo beans, tomato sauce, and half of the onion, garlic, and carrot mixture in a food processor. Blend until a 'dough' forms. It is okay if some of the pasta and beans are not completelty smooth; a few pea-sized pieces will add texture to the burger. Place all the other ingredients in a bowl and, a little bit at a time, fold them into the bean and pasta dough until all ingredients are incorporated. You might have some of the quinoa mixture left over, which we recommend saving for snacking. Form the patties into hamburger-sized disks and let them set in the refrigerator for about 30 minutes. You can either lightly (and gently) grill or bake these patties in a very hot oven. We find baking the burgers works best on a generously oiled baking sheet or glass dish, with the oven turned up to 425-450°F. Flip the burgers after 8-10 minutes, and bake them until a golden brown crust forms on each side, roughly 15-20 minutes total.

Prep Time 1 hour and 45 minutes (this includes the resting time in the refrigerator).

Serves 6.

Notes

Three Cheese Lasagna with Basil and Tomato

With today's numerous low-fat and fat-free versions of traditional high-fat products, eating a healthy diet is easy. This lasagna allows you the decadence of a cheesy favorite without the dairy fat that can compromise your health. You can sprinkle cooked spinach in between the layers for additional antioxidant benefits. If for some reason your local stores do not have the fat-free versions of these cheese products, try soy or rice cheese, or skip to the next recipe—but don't gamble with your health by consuming the regular high-fat versions.

SHOPPING LIST
1 pound lasagna noodles, whole wheat or spinach
1-1/2 pints nonfat ricotta cheese or 12 ounces soft tofu
1 pound nonfat mozzarella cheese
1/2 cup nonfat Parmesan
2 tablespoons basil, chopped
1/2 cup egg whites
1-1/2 pints tomato sauce

PREPARATION
Cook the noodles using the directions on the package and completely drain them of liquid. In a small bowl, mix the ricotta cheese with the basil and egg whites. In a large rectangular baking pan, ladle in tomato sauce to just cover the bottom. Layer the noodles followed by more sauce and the mozzarella cheese. Add another layer of noodles, and spoon and smooth the ricotta cheese mixture over the top. Add more sauce, and repeat the layers twice. Over the final layer of noodles, add more sauce and sprinkle in the Parmesan cheese. Cover the lasagna with parchment and then aluminum foil. (Parchment paper will prevent the foil's metallic taste from entering the lasagna). Bake the dish for 40 minutes in a 400°F, oven. Remove the foil and wax paper and bake the dish uncovered for 10

minutes. Remove the dish from the oven, and let it rest for 10 minutes before serving.

Prep time 1/2 hour. *Total time* 2 hours.

Serves 6.

Notes

Vegan Lasagna With Spiced Tofu and Spinach

If you want a cheese-free version of lasagna, the following recipe will satisfy your craving for baked pasta. We've added chickpeas to increase the overall fiber and included a soy-based cheese substitute for those who are lactose intolerant or who don't eat dairy products for social or religious reasons.

SHOPPING LIST
1 onion, chopped
4 garlic cloves, minced
1 28-ounce can crushed tomatoes
1 6-ounce can tomato paste
2 teaspoons basil, chopped
1 teaspoon oregano, chopped
1/2 teaspoon thyme, chopped
1 teaspoon fennel seeds, ground
1/2 teaspoon black pepper
1 tablespoon olive oil
Salt, to taste
1 pound firm tofu mashed
1/2 teaspoon salt
1/8 teaspoon nutmeg
1/8 teaspoon cinnamon
1/2 teaspoon black pepper
1 pound cooked spinach, chopped and pressed of water
1 15-ounce can chickpeas, drained and processed smooth,
    with a dash of water or olive oil to process
1/2 cup fresh dill, chopped
1 8-ounce package vegan soy or rice cheese, grated
1 pound package lasagna noodles

PREPARATION
Cook the noodles using the directions on the package and completely drain them of liquid. Heat olive oil in a large skillet

213

and sauté the onion and garlic until tender. Add the tomatoes, tomato paste, herbs, and spices. Simmer the sauce for 15 minutes. Preheat the oven to 350°F. Combine the mashed tofu, salt, nutmeg, cinnamon, and black pepper. Set aside. Add the dill to the processed chickpeas and mix. To assemble the lasagna spread 1 cup of the sauce in a 9 x 12 inch pan. Cover the bottom with a layer of noodles. Working in layers, alternate a layer of tofu mixture and spinach, a layer of pasta, tomato sauce and a layer of the vegan cheese and chickpea mixture. Repeat the layering twice. End with the noodles and a layer of sauce. Cover with wax paper and foil and bake for 30 minutes. Let stand for 10 minutes before serving. Garnish with torn fresh basil leaves or chopped parsley.

Preparation time 1-1/4 hours.

Serves 10-12.

Notes

Summer Zucchini, Tomato, and Bean Casserole with Parmesan

Vegetables that grow and fruit in the same season tend to taste better together: tomatoes with zucchini; tomatoes with eggplant; and tomatoes with basil compliment each other and offer us a culinary canvas of summer's bounty. In this casserole we present four ingredients, which thrive together: zucchini, tomato, shelling beans, and basil. The first version of this recipe is easy to prepare, leaving plenty of time to do other things in the kitchen before it is ready. The second version is more labor intensive and takes less time from start to finish.

SHOPPING LIST

3 tablespoons olive oil
1 cup onion, chopped
8 garlic cloves, minced
3 cups zucchini, medium diced
1-1/2 cups plum tomatoes, chopped with juice
1-1/2 cups cooked mixed beans
   (red kidney, chickpea, northern white)
1/4 cup fresh basil, torn
2 teaspoons fresh thyme, chopped
1/2 cup grated low or nonfat Parmesan cheese
Salt and black pepper, to taste

PREPARATION

Version 1
Preheat the oven to 350°F. In a large bowl, thoroughly mix all ingredients, except the cheese. Place the mixture in a casserole dish coasted with olive oil. Bake the casserole for 35 minutes, rotating the dish at least once to ensure even cooking. Remove the casserole from the oven and distribute Parmesan over the top. Return the dish to the oven, and continue baking until the

215

cheese browns. Remove the casserole from the oven, let it set for 5 minutes, and serve.

Prep time 1-1/2 hours.

Serves 6.

Version 2

Heat olive oil in a large skillet, add the zucchini, and sauté until browned. Remove the zucchini from the skillet and set aside. Preheat the broiler. Add the garlic and onions to the skillet and cook them until translucent. Add the tomatoes, herbs, and beans. Bring the mixture to a simmer for about 7 minutes. Mix in the cheese and zucchini and place the mixture in an oiled baking dish. Place the casserole under the broiler until the cheese browns. Remove the dish from the broiler, let it set for 5 minutes and serve.

Prep time 45 minutes.

Serves 6.

Notes

Meatless Meatloaf

Okay, so this meatloaf doesn't actually contain any meat, but we've learned that herbs, spices, and aromatic vegetables combined with a meat-like texture can get us close to the traditional meatloaf. We've suggested a product like Boca in this recipe, but in today's supermarkets several companies sell soy or gluten-based ground beef and sausage substitutes.

SHOPPING LIST
1 12-ounce package ground soy or gluten like Boca or
   Morningstar Farms or an organic alternative.
1-1/2 cups cooked lentils
1 onion, chopped
3 celery stalks, chopped
2 carrots, chopped
2 garlic cloves, minced
1 tablespoon basil, chopped
1 teaspoon oregano, chopped
2 tablespoons olive oil
3-4 egg whites
Salt and pepper, to taste

Garnish
1/2 cup marinara sauce
1 tablespoon parsley, chopped

PREPARATION
Sauté the onion, garlic, celery, and carrot in olive oil until tender. In a bowl, combine the ground soy or gluten, lentils, vegetables, and herbs. Beat the egg whites until slightly frothy, and knead them into the mixture. Coat a baking dish with olive oil. Transfer the mixture to the oiled baking dish and press the mixture to form a loaf. Bake at 350°F, for 30 minutes. Garnish with marinara sauce and parsley.

217

Prep time 1 hour. *Total time* 1-1/2 hours.

Serves 4.

Notes

Crab Cakes

Mayonnaise and sour cream are used to bind most crab cakes that you buy in restaurants. The cakes are almost always pan-fried and finished in the oven. In the following recipe, we've used aioli and egg whites to bind our cakes, and replaced frying with a straightforward oven bake. A high oven should mimic the intense heat that frying creates and evenly brown the cakes.

SHOPPING LIST
15 ounces jumbo lump blue crabmeat
1 cup fine breadcrumbs
2 ounces egg whites
1/2 cup homemade aioli or olive oil mayonnaise
1/2 teaspoon Worcestershire sauce
1 teaspoon Dijon mustard
2 teaspoons lemon zest, chopped
2 teaspoons lemon juice
1/2 teaspoon salt
1/2 teaspoon pepper
2 tablespoons fresh parsley, finely chopped
2 tablespoons fresh chives, thinly sliced

PREPARATION
Examine the crabmeat for small pieces of shell. If you use canned crabmeat, be sure to squeeze out any excess moisture from the meat before placing it in a large bowl. In a separate medium-sized bowl, whisk the aioli into the whites, add the Worcestershire sauce, mustard, lemon juice and zest, salt, and pepper. Place half of the breadcrumbs on top of the crabmeat in a large bowl. Pour half the egg mixture on top of this and gently mix together. If you like your cakes dry, add more breadcrumbs; if you like them wet, add more egg. Mix in the parsley and chives. Form into 6–8 balls. Pat them slightly flat with your hand to form "pucks." Use the remaining

breadcrumbs to coat the cakes and place them on a large plate or baking sheet. Refrigerate the cakes for one hour. Lightly oil a baking sheet and lay the crab on the sheet. Preheat the oven to 450°F,. Bake the cakes until golden brown on both sides and cooked through. Garnish with a dab of aioli or olive oil mayonnaise and a lemon wedge.

Prep time 45 minutes.

Serves 6.

Notes

Fish Stew with Saffron, Tomato, and Fennel

Fragrant fennel, garlic zing, the vibrant acidity of tomatoes, and saffron's delicate sweetness create the base for this fish stew. While we've provided a classic Mediterranean fish stew in many ways with the following recipe, we've swerved by adding butternut squash; we find butternut goes surprising well with tomato.

SHOPPING LIST
2 tablespoons olive oil
2 large onions, diced
6 garlic cloves, minced
1/2 teaspoon fennel seeds, ground
1/2 teaspoon saffron threads, dissolved in warm water
1 28-ounce can peeled whole tomatoes, drained and chopped
  (*reserve liquid*)
1 quart fish stock
1 cup fennel bulb, diced
1 small butternut squash, peeled, seeded, and large diced
1 teaspoon orange zest
1 teaspoon lemon zest
1 bay leaf
1-1/2 pounds cod, halibut, or bass, cut into chunks
  roughly 2 inches by 2 inches
1/2 teaspoon freshly ground black pepper
1/4 cup fresh parsley, chopped
Salt, to taste

PREPARATION
Heat the olive oil in a large pot, add the onions, fennel bulb, and garlic; cook the vegetables until soft and translucent. Add the saffron, fennel seeds, tomatoes and their juice, bay leaf, and zest. Simmer uncovered for ten minutes. Add the fish stock, and bring the stew to a low boil. Add the squash, bring

the stew to a simmer, and cook the squash ¾ of the way before adding the cod. Cook the fish on a low simmer, until just set. Be careful not to overcook the fish. Serve the stew immediately. If you cannot serve the stew right away, remove the fish from the hot liquid and set it on a plate to cool. Garnish the fragrant stew with chopped parsley and a drizzle of extra virgin olive oil, and serve.

Prep time 1-1/4 hours.

Serves 6.

Notes

Monkfish with Savory Ginger Yogurt, Carrot, and Pistachio

Monkfish braised in a tangy ginger-yogurt sauce provides a hearty base for this savory dish. If you cannot find monkfish, try the following recipe with shrimp or squid.

SHOPPING LIST
2 pounds monkfish, cleaned and cut into bite-sized pieces
   (about 1" inch by 1 inch)
2 large white onions, sliced
2' by 2' piece of fresh ginger, peeled
3 garlic cloves, peeled
1/4 cup lemon juice
1 teaspoon salt (more or less, depending on taste)
2 tablespoons olive oil for sautéing
1/8 teaspoon whole cloves, ground
1/2 tablespoon black peppercorns, ground
1/2 tablespoon fennel seeds, ground
1/4 tablespoon mustard seeds, ground
1/4 tablespoon coriander seeds, ground
1/4 tablespoon cumin seeds, ground
1 cup plain nonfat yogurt
1-1/2 cups brown basmati rice
1/3 cup fish or vegetable stock
1/2 teaspoon saffron threads
1/2 cup golden raisins
1/3 cup shredded carrot
1/4 cup pistachios

PREPARATION
Preheat the oven to 375°F.

    Quarter one onion and put it into a food processor with the garlic, ginger, and lemon juice; puree the vegetables until smooth. Pour the mixture into a bowl. Thinly slice one onion, and slowly sauté it with all of the spices until the onion is soft and the spices fragrant. Remove the spicy onions from the heat, and stir them into the yogurt and ginger-lemon-onion mixture until all the ingredients are incorporated. Cover and refrigerate.

Meanwhile, bring 4 cups salted water to a boil, add the rice, and simmer for 20 minutes. Drain the rice in a strainer.

In a decorative baking dish, first add the monkfish, season the fish with salt, then add the yogurt sauce, and finish the dish with a layer of rice. In a small pan, bring the stock and saffron to a simmer. Remove the pan from the heat and let stand for 2 minutes. Pour the liquid in streaks over the rice, and sprinkle raisins over the rice. Cover the dish first in parchment paper and then in aluminum foil, and bake it in the oven for 45 minutes to 1 hour, or until the fish is cooked through. Be sure to rotate the baking dish halfway through to ensure even cooking. Garnish with shredded carrots and pistachios.

Prep time 30 minutes. *Total time* 1-1 ½ hours.

Serves 6.

Notes

Bayou Shrimp Stew

This shrimp stew establishes the rich taste of shrimp from the bottom up by using shells to create a flavorful base. We've added red and yellow peppers to the classic trinity of green peppers, onions, and celery to enhance the piquant kick of this regional stew. If you like crab, add a few ounces of cooked crabmeat to the stew about 2-3 minutes after adding the shrimp to heat it through.

SHOPPING LIST
2 tablespoons olive oil
3/4 cup whole wheat flour
1 pound medium shrimp in the shells
3 cups water
1 cup white wine
1 bay leaf
2-1/2 cups onions, sliced
2 cups celery, sliced
1 cup green bell pepper, diced
1 cup yellow or red bell pepper, diced
1 cup scallions, sliced
1 large carrot, diced
4 garlic cloves, minced
1/8 teaspoon red pepper flakes
1 teaspoon thyme
1 cup fresh parsley, chopped
4 cups cooked brown rice
Salt, to taste

PREPARATION
Make a roux: heat the oil in a heavy pan, slowly stir in the flour, and cook on low to medium heat until it just begins to brown. Reduce the heat and continue to cook the roux, stirring often, for about 10 minutes.

Peel and de-vein the shrimp. Save the shells. In a saucepan boil 3 cups of water and 1 cup of white wine. Add shrimp shells and bay leaf and cook for 40 minutes. Remove the shells and reserve the stock. Sauté the onions, garlic, green peppers, carrots, red pepper flakes, and celery in olive oil until tender. Season this base with salt and pepper. Add the roux and stir into the base. Once the roux is incorporated, slowly stir in the reserved shrimp stock. Add the red or yellow pepper and thyme and check the stew for seasoning. Simmer for 30 minutes, stirring the pot occasionally to make sure the vegetables that have settled on the bottom get released. Add the shrimp to the stew and simmer for 5 minutes. Garnish the stew with scallions and parsley, and serve the fragrant mix over warm brown rice.

Prep time 1-1/2 hours.

Serves 4.

Notes

Roasted Cod with Citrus Emulsion

This bright unctuous sauce plays against the cod's full flavor and lean texture. Try varying the citrus in this recipe with Japanese yuzu, key lime, or blood orange juice. (We love the color that blood orange juice brings to the plate). If you cannot find fresh cod, substitute halibut or sole. You can use the citrus emulsion as a dip for lobster or crabmeat. Chop a handful of chervil and stir it into the sauce before dipping.

SHOPPING LIST
Sauce
2 tablespoons fresh squeezed orange juice
3 tablespoons fresh squeezed lemon juice
2 teaspoons lemon zest
1 teaspoon dry mustard
5 tablespoons extra virgin olive oil
Sea salt and white pepper, to taste

Fish
2 pounds cod fillets
1/2 teaspoon white pepper
2 scallions, sliced thin
Skin of one lemon, sliced in thin strips

PREPARATION
Preheat the oven to 400°F. Sprinkle olive oil on a baking dish large enough to hold the fish in a single layer. Meanwhile, start whisking the juice, mustard, lemon zest, salt, and pepper, and slowly add the olive oil until emulsified. Set aside. Lay the thin strips of lemon in the oiled baking dish. Rinse the fish, pat it dry, and place it in the baking dish on top of the lemon strips. Season the fish with salt. Bake the fish until it just begins to set and flake, about 8-12 minutes. Transfer the fish to a warm

serving platter. Sprinkle the lemon strips around the platter. Spoon the sauce over the fish, garnish with scallions, and serve.

Prep time 45 minutes.

Serves 4.

Notes

Breaded Chicken Breast With Herbs and Spices

We can't beat fried chicken, but the following recipe provides a crispy crust and tender juicy chicken breast without the weight and regret of the fried version. If you have time, try seasoning your chicken breast with salt 6-8 hours before beginning the recipe as it will help tenderize the meat and make it juicy and well seasoned.

SHOPPING LIST
4 chicken breasts, de-boned and skinned
1/2 cup breadcrumbs
1 tablespoon powdered garlic
1 tablespoon oregano
1 tablespoon basil
1/2 tablespoon coriander
1/8 teaspoon cayenne pepper (optional)
1/2 cup egg whites
1 teaspoon tomato paste
Salt and pepper, to taste

PREPARATION
Preheat the oven to 400°F. Wash and dry the chicken and remove all the fat. Mix the breadcrumbs with the herbs, spices, and salt in a shallow bowl. In another shallow bowl, whisk the egg whites and tomato paste. Coat the chicken with the whites, and then with the breadcrumbs. Put the chicken in a baking dish or pan coated with olive oil. Bake the chicken in the oven until just cooked through. Some people will want to sprinkle a little salt on the chicken before it is served. Baked chicken needs a good dipping sauce; depending on your taste, you might try dipping the tender chicken in our pesto, tapenade, or aioli sauces—of course, sometimes nothing beats a good swim in ketchup.

Prep time 45 minutes.

Serves 4-6.

Notes

Breaded Chicken Breast with Herbs and Spices, Grape-nut Variation

Similar to the previous recipe, this version of baked chicken is made with Grape-Nuts cereal.

SHOPPING LIST
1 pound chicken tenders
1/2 cup Grape-Nuts, crushed finely
1 tablespoon garlic, minced
1 tablespoon oregano, chopped
1 tablespoon basil, chopped
1/2 tablespoon coriander
1/2 cup egg whites
Salt and pepper, to taste

PREPARATION
Preheat the oven to 400°F. Wash and dry the chicken and remove all the fat. Mix the seasoned Grape-Nuts cereal with the herbs, spices, and salt in a shallow bowl. In another shallow bowl whisk the egg whites. Coat the chicken with the whites, and then with the Grape-Nuts cereal. Put the chicken in a baking dish or pan coated with olive oil. Bake the chicken in the oven until just cooked through.

Prep time 45 minutes.

Serves 4.

Notes

Wine and Herb Poached Chicken

By poaching proteins, you avoid using oils and fats in the cooking process altogether. We avoid frying and pan-frying as heating oil at very high temperatures can cause carcinogens that the outer chicken or fish flesh will easily absorb. Poaching allows the subtle flavors of any meat, fish, or egg to surface without the influence of heated oil.

SHOPPING LIST
4 chicken breasts, de-boned and skinned
2 cups water
2 cups white wine (Sauvignon Blanc or Pinot Grigio)
5 sprigs fresh or 1 tablespoon dry thyme
1 small onion, quartered
1/2 teaspoon fresh rosemary, chopped
1 bay leaf
Salt, to taste

PREPARATION
In a wide stockpot, bring the water, salt, wine, onion, and herbs to a boil. Cook the poaching liquid uncovered for 5 minutes. Bring the liquid down to a strong simmer, and add the chicken breast. Your poaching liquid should be at a low simmer while the chicken cooks. When they are cooked through, remove the breasts from the bath, dry, and serve with a green onion relish, green olive tapenade, or pesto sauce.

Prep time 35 minutes.

Serves 4.

Notes

Salmon En Papillote With Fresh Dill and Lemon

Cooking "en papillote," a French phrase for "in the package," allows each portion to gently cook and sweat in its own juices. By sealing salmon in little envelopes with aromatic vegetables, lemon, and herbs, the fish becomes delicately infused with those aromatics. Another method that avoids heating oil to dangerous temperatures, en papillote can be used to cook almost any fish or poultry, although fish that tastes best rare, such as ahi tuna, would not be a good choice for en papillote.

SHOPPING LIST
1-3 pounds whole fresh cleaned salmon (head and tail removed)
1/2 cup of fresh dill, chopped
1-2 large lemons, thinly sliced
1-2 teaspoons olive oil
Salt and white pepper, to taste

PREPARATION
Preheat the oven to 350° F. Wash and dry the salmon, and season the flesh with dill, salt, white pepper, and olive oil. Cut the fillet into individual portions, about 5-6 ounces per person. Place each salmon portion in a wax paper envelope. (We recommend using unbleached brown wax paper.) Lay a thin slice of lemon on the top and bottom of each portion. Close and tightly seal the wax paper. Place the envelopes in a baking dish or pan, and bake them for 6-10 minutes. Check a package to see how the salmon is cooking—ideally, salmon should be cooked medium-rare with the center of the fish barley set. If you like your fish cooked more, just allow it to cook longer, but do not overcook the fish. Remove the envelopes from the oven. Lay the salmon on a serving dish lined with parsley or dill. A sauce of nonfat yogurt with dill and salted and diced cucumbers

works great for a hot summer day sauce. Our salsa verde also pairs well with the salmon.

Prep time 1-1/2 hours.

Serves 4- 10.

Notes

Whole "Grilled" Salmon With Fresh Herbs

While the following recipe details how to cook a whole salmon on the grill, you can use the same method to cook almost any whole fish, just make sure to adjust the cooking times.

SHOPPING LIST
1 whole fresh salmon

Dry Marinade
1 tablespoon salt
1/4 cup brown sugar
1 tablespoon white pepper

Cooking Broth
6 cloves garlic, minced
1 ounce ginger, peeled and sliced into quarter-sized pieces
6 green onions, cleaned and cut lengthwise
4 carrots, cleaned, peeled, and cut thin lengthwise
4 celery stalks, cleaned and cut lengthwise
Bouquet of fresh herbs, discussed below
1 large, Meyer lemon, juiced and peeled
2 cups water
Salt and white pepper, to taste

Herb Bouquets
4-5 large sprigs basil
5 small sprigs oregano
5 small sprigs thyme
8 large sprigs parsley
1 large sprig rosemary

PREPARATION
Scale, wash, and pat the salmon dry. Mix the dry marinade and wipe it into the salmon cavity. Refrigerate the marinating

235

salmon for 4 to 8 hours.

Remove the salmon from the refrigerator about ½ hour before cooking to bring it to room temperature. Dry off the exterior of the fish and wipe out the cavity, removing any loose marinade. (Do not rinse the fish again as it will absorb some of the rinse water.)

Get the grill very hot, and reduce the grill setting to low or rake the coals so that they are dispersed enough for low heat. If you have a long enough oven-proof baking dish for the salmon, use it to hold the cooking broth and salmon. If you do not have a long baking dish, form a large sheet of aluminum foil into a baking sheet sufficiently large enough to hold the fish, liquid, herbs, and vegetables. Line this baking sheet with parchment paper so that it completely covers the aluminum foil. (Try not to let your food come in direct contact with aluminum foil—it can give your food a metallic taste and react with acidic products.) Pour one cup of the water with the lemon juice onto the aluminum foil/parchment-lined baking sheet. Add the fish to the baking sheet, and then add the sliced vegetables and herbs. The herbs and vegetables should be spaced evenly around the fish. At this point close the grill and wait. Replenish the cooking broth as it evaporates.

Cooking time for this dish is an art, dependent on the size of the fish and the heat of your grill. The objective is for the side of the fish facing the grill to be mostly cooked when the fish is carefully turned onto the other side. This is done when the skin on the grill facing side could be easily removed from the fish, approximately 45 minutes. The second side will be done when the skin on the second side is easily loosened from the fish, about 30 minutes.

When cooked, carefully remove the skin from the upward facing side of the fish. Remove the fish from the "pan" gently using several wide spatulas and place it on a serving platter skin side down. Remove the remaining skin from the fish. Another way to remove the fish from the foil is to first remove the cooking broth, herbs, and vegetables from the foil and place the serving platter over the skinned side of the fish. The platter, fish, and foil are then turned over and the skin from the second side is removed. Garnish the fish with fresh herbs and serve. The flesh will easily lift off the salmon with a wide spatula.

Although the grilled salmon can be frozen, it doesn't seem to taste as good when de-frosted, so send any leftovers home with your guests. By the way, the residual broth is delicious for use as a soup or sauce base.

Prep time 2 hours. *Total time* 6-10 hours.

Serves 6-8.

Notes

On The Side

Savory Rice With Shiitake Mushrooms

Rich in the Shiitake's earthy flavor, this high fiber side-dish pairs with roasted chicken, turkey, or fall vegetables. Try using the savory rice as a stuffing for game hen or rabbit.

SHOPPING LIST
1 tablespoon olive oil
1 medium onion, finely chopped
3 garlic cloves, minced
1/4 pound fresh Shiittake mushrooms, sliced
   (for dried mushrooms rehydrate in hot water, drain,
   and then thinly slice)
3 cups chicken stock
1 cup oat bran
1 cup cooked long grain brown rice
Salt and black pepper, to taste

Garnish
Parsley, chopped
Extra virgin olive oil

PREPARATION
Heat the oil in a large saucepan over medium to low heat. Add the onion and cook for one minute. Add the garlic, season the vegetables, and cook for four minutes. Push the mixture to the outer edges of the pan and raise the heat to medium. Add the mushrooms and stir the vegetable mix until it begins to brown. Stir in the chicken stock and scrape the sides and bottom of the pan. Bring the stock to a low boil. Stir in the oat bran and constantly whisk the ingredients until the mixture thickens, usually about 2-3 minutes. With a wooden spoon, stir the cooked rice into the bran mixture. Transfer the mixture to a serving dish. Garnish with parsley and a drizzle of extra virgin olive oil.

Prep time 1-1/2 hours. If rice is precooked, 45 minutes.

Serves 4.

Notes

Wilted Escarole and Millet with Roasted Garlic

The following recipe calls for escarole, a member of the chicory family that has broad and tender leaves which readily absorb flavors. If you can't find escarole, try this recipe with kale or collards greens, but be sure to adjust the cooking time for these greens, as they take longer to cook. If you do not appreciate the flavor or texture of millet, use white navy beans.

SHOPPING LIST
1 pound tender escarole
2 large heads garlic, roasted
2 cups millet, cooked
2 tablespoons extra virgin olive oil
Salt and black pepper, to taste

PREPARATION
Preheat oven to 375°F. Remove the base from the escarole, then rinse and dry. Bring a large pot of salted water to a boil. Submerge the greens in the water, and cook for 1-3 minutes, or until wilted and tender. Drain and spread the greens in a single layer on a baking pan to cool. Once cooled, squeeze the escarole to remove as much moisture as possible. Depending on the size of the leaves, you might want to chop the escarole leaves so they're easier to eat. In the meantime, place the garlic in a small baking dish and cook at 350-375°F, for 30 minutes. Remove from the oven and cool. Squeeze the garlic cloves out of their skins, and mix them into the millet. Mash the cloves with a fork, and season the mixture to taste with salt and pepper. In a large bowl, combine the escarole and millet and mix until evenly dispersed. Serve with a drizzle of extra virgin olive oil.

Prep time 45 minutes.

Serves 6.

Quinoa Timbales

An ancient Incan grain with a high amount of quality protein, quinoa acts as a great side dish for poultry and fish, but it can stand on its own as the main protein source in a meal. You can enjoy the light fluffy texture of quinoa by not overcooking the grain; overcooked quinoa becomes mushy when the grain blows out of its tight structure. By packing quinoa into timbales, you can highlight the grain's visual appeal and distinct texture.

SHOPPING LIST
1 cup quinoa
1 medium onion, small diced
1 tablespoon olive oil
1/2 teaspoon ground cumin
1/8 teaspoon cinnamon
1/4 teaspoon turmeric
1 teaspoon lemon zest, chopped
1 2/3 cups vegetable stock
1/3 cup organic golden raisins
1/4 cup tomatoes, chopped and drained
Salt and pepper, to taste

Garnish
3 tablespoons fresh parsley, chopped

PREPARATION
In a heavy-bottom pan, sauté the onion in olive oil until tender and translucent. Add the spices and quinoa, stir, and cook for 2 minutes. Add the stock, tomatoes, raisins, salt, and pepper and bring the mixture to a simmer. Cover the pot and cook the quinoa until it absorbs the liquid. Remove the pan from the heat and stir in the parsley. Divide the quinoa among 6 lightly oiled timbale molds, and firmly pack each timbale. Invert the

timbales onto individual plates or a platter, garnish with parsley and extra virgin olive oil, and serve.

Prep time 1/2 hour.

Serves 6.

Notes

Artichokes à la Micheline

Artichokes have some of the same polyphenols found in green tea. Whole artichokes make a dramatic addition to any meal as an appealing appetizer or lunchtime snack. We've adjusted Rose and Sara's Sicilian family recipe to include fresh herbs, garlic, and lemon zest, which increases the overall antioxidant power of the dish. The steamed artichokes can be served cold and cut as part of an antipasti platter. If serving cut, be sure to remove the thistles that form at the base of the leaves.

SHOPPING LIST
4–6 medium artichokes
2 tablespoons lemon juice
1 tablespoon lemon zest
1/2 cup breadcrumbs
4-5 garlic cloves, minced
1 tablespoon oregano, chopped
1 tablespoon basil, chopped
1 tablespoon coriander, ground
1 tablespoon olive oil
1/4 cup grated Romano cheese (optional)
Salt, to taste

Garnish
2 tablespoons parsley, chopped
2 tablespoons extra virgin olive oil

PREPARATION
Wash and dry the artichokes. Trim about 1/2 inch off the top of each artichoke. Drizzle the tops with lemon juice. Spread the leaves open and place the artichokes in a large pot. Fill the pot with 1-1/2 inches of vegetable stock. Sprinkle the breadcrumbs, lemon zest, fresh herbs, salt, and cheese over the tops of the artichokes. Make sure the ingredients settle among the leaves.

Drizzle olive oil over the artichokes and cover the pot. Cook the artichokes on low heat until the base of the leaves are tender. Lift the 'chokes from the pot and serve. Garnish with a drizzle of extra virgin olive oil and chopped parsley. Serve hot or cold.

Prep time 1-1/2 hours.

Serves 4–6.

Notes

Grilled Vegetables With Balsamic and Fresh Basil

Grilling desiccates and concentrates the flavors of ripe vegetables. We find marinating vegetables in balsamic vinegar, olive oil, and fresh herbs helps draw the sweetness out and provides an aromatic background to the grill char.

SHOPPING LIST
1 medium eggplant, sliced lengthwise
2 large onions, peeled with root base intact, sliced
1 large bell pepper, trimmed, cleaned of seeds, and cut in large strips
4 fingerling potatoes, cleaned and cut thin lengthwise
2 leek stalks, trimmed, cut in half, and washed under cold running water
2 fennel stalks, cleaned and cut in thirds with root base intact
2 carrots, peeled and cut lengthwise
2-4 large oyster, porcini, or portobello mushrooms, brushed clean, and depending on size, cut in half or left whole (if you use portobellos, be sure to cut or scrape the dark gills off— they will stain the other vegetables, and their texture is less than desirable)
3 tablespoons extra virgin olive oil
5 garlic cloves, minced
2 tablespoons balsamic vinegar
1/4 cup fresh oregano, chopped
1/4 cup rosemary, chopped fine
1/4 cup fresh basil leaves, torn
Salt and pepper, to taste

PREPARATION
Clean and prepare the vegetables and herbs as suggested. Whisk the following ingredients into the olive oil: garlic, oregano, rosemary, salt, and pepper. Place the vegetables in a large bowl or deep pan, and pour the seasoned oil over the

vegetables. Toss the vegetables to make sure the marinade has evenly coated each surface. Let the vegetables marinate for 30 minutes. Drain the vegetables, season, and grill until tender, marked, and *lightly* browned on both sides. Be attentive to each vegetable group: the cooking time can vary greatly between each ingredient. If a grill is not available, broil the vegetables in a hot oven. Pour the remaining marinade over the grilled vegetables, and garnish with fresh torn basil.

Prep time 30 minutes. *Total time* 1-1/4 hours.

Serves 4.

Notes

Red Pepper Stuffed with Millet and Mint

A grain high in B vitamins, millet tends to thrive in arid climates with poor soil. Its high nutritional content has made it a staple in Africa and many parts of Asia.

The grain's mild flavor acts to absorb the sweetness of roasted peppers in this recipe.

SHOPPING LIST

1 cup millet
2 cups vegetable stock, plus 2 tablespoons for cooking
   the peppers
1 medium red onion, finely chopped
2 celery stalks, finely chopped
2 garlic cloves, minced
1 cup corn
1 tablespoon fresh mint, chopped
2 teaspoons lemon zest, grated
1-1/2 teaspoons fresh oregano, chopped
1 teaspoon black pepper, ground
4 medium red bell peppers, tops removed, seeded, and ribbed
3-4 tablespoons extra virgin olive oil
2 tablespoons fresh lemon juice
Salt, to taste

PREPARATION

Preheat an oven to 375 °F. Wash the millet by placing it in a fine mesh strainer, and rinsing it under cold running water. Bring the vegetable stock to a boil and stir in the millet. Reduce the heat after the millet/stock comes to a boil. Cover the pot and gently simmer the millet/stock for 20 minutes. Turn the burner off and let the millet steam for 15 minutes. Remove the cover and let the millet cool for 15 to 20 minutes before fluffing it with a fork. Sauté the onion, celery, garlic, and corn in olive oil until tender. Mix the millet and vegetables. Add the mint, lemon zest, oregano, and season to taste with ground pepper and salt. Cut a very thin slice off the bottom of each red pepper, taking care not to pierce through the flesh into the pepper cup. Stuff each pepper with the millet mixture. Brush or drizzle the top of each pepper with a bit of the olive oil. Place the peppers in a rectangular baking pan, just large enough to hold them. Add stock to the baking dish, up to 1 inch. Place the dish in the center rack of the oven and cook for 30-40 minutes, or until the red peppers cook through. In a small bowl, whisk together the remaining oil and lemon juice. Spoon a bit of this dressing into each pepper before serving, and garnish with a little mint.

Prep time 1 hour and 20 minutes.

Serves 4.

Notes

Basic Recipe for Savory Greens with Garlic

Throughout the Mediterranean, it is common practice for the women to walk the roadsides and fields collecting wild greens. Rose still remembers her mother and her other Sicilian relatives gathering greens from Pennsylvanian roadsides during her childhood. You can use any of the following greens for this basic recipe: dandelion, rapini, spinach, escarole, turnip greens, collards, kale, arugula, or mustard. A quick and easy way to incorporate more greens into your diet is to cook a big batch on the weekend and use them throughout the week mixed into pasta, grains, or beans. If you like spicy heat in your greens, add crushed red pepper flakes to the pan with the garlic; if you can find smoked peppers, crush and add them to the garlic for a flavor reminiscent of bacon or smoked ham hocks.

SHOPPING LIST
2 pounds of greens
1 tablespoon olive oil
3-6 garlic cloves, minced or ½ cup shallots, minced
1-1/2 cups vegetable or chicken stock (optional)
Salt and black pepper, to taste

PREPARATION
Trim and wash the greens in cold water. Depending on the size of the greens, you may need to tear or chop them into mouth-sized pieces. In olive oil, quickly bloom the garlic or shallots until fragrant and add the greens. When you cook a tougher green, you might need to add stock to the pan—sturdy greens such as kale, collards, and some rapinis will most likely need stock added. Spinach and arugula will need to be drained of their juices before serving. When the greens are tender, remove them from the heat, drain, and serve either hot, cold, or at room temperature. Garnish the greens with a drizzle of extra virgin olive oil.

Prep time 20 minutes.

Serves 6–8.

Notes

Tomato Garlic Bread

When tomato season hits, pluck your best homegrown or go to the farmers' market for this simple appetizer which highlights the sweetness and acidity of ripe tomatoes.

SHOPPING LIST
1 baguette
6 –8 large garlic cloves, minced
2 tablespoons olive oil
1/4 cup Parmesan cheese (or nonfat shredded mozzarella or
    provolone)
1/4 teaspoon fresh basil, torn
1/4 teaspoon fresh oregano, chopped
2-3 small slicing tomatoes
Ground black pepper and sea salt, to taste

PREPARATION
Cut baguette in half and slice both halves lengthwise, drizzle the bread with olive oil, and spread the garlic evenly over the surface. Toast the bread for one minute under your broiler, or until the garlic blooms and becomes aromatic. Add the cheese, and broil for 2-4 minutes, or until a golden crust forms (check constantly to avoid burning!) Cover the surface with juicy tomato slices and finish with basil, oregano, ground pepper, and sea salt.

Prep time 15 minutes.

Serves 4.

Notes

Oven-Baked Potatoes

A trouble-free way to reap the health benefits of the potato: abstain from adding high fat sour cream, butter, and bacon once you cut open the steaming vegetable. In the following recipe, we list possible alternatives to the traditional toppings.

SHOPPING LIST
6 medium Russet or sweet potatoes, scrubbed
Salt and pepper
Parsley

PREPARATION
Wash the potatoes and prick them with a fork. Place the potatoes on an oven rack in a 400°F, oven. Bake them until done, approximately 45 minutes. White potatoes can be served plain or with aioli, salsa, pesto, nonfat sour cream, yogurt, scallions, chives, or a drizzle of olive oil. Sweet potatoes can be served plain or with chopped nuts, brown sugar, fruit compote, or chopped herbs. Season to taste with salt and pepper.

Prep time 5 minutes. *Total time* 50 minutes.

Serves 6.

Notes

Oven-Browned Potatoes

SHOPPING LIST

6 medium Yukon gold, fingerling, or red potatoes,
   scrubbed and quartered
1 teaspoon each chopped parsley, oregano, basil,
   and minced garlic
Salt and pepper, to taste

PREPARATION

Preheat your oven to 350°F.

Quarter and place the potatoes in a baking dish that has been
lightly coated in olive oil. Season the potatoes with salt and
pepper and bake until cooked through. In large bowl, toss the
potatoes with fresh herbs. If you would like to add garlic, swirl
minced garlic in the hot baking pan until bloomed and fragrant
and scrape it into the potato bowl. Toss the potatoes to ensure
the garlic is evenly distributed, and serve.

Prep time 5 minutes. *Total time* 40 minutes.

Serves 6.

Notes

Onions Agrodolce

Another Sicilian culinary contribution, "agrodolce" means "sour" and "sweet." The basic sauce requires a reduction of vinegar and sugar until it becomes a syrup that coats the ingredients. A popular version of agrodolce slowly braises cipollini onions in aged Balsamic vinegar until tender and swimming in piquant syrup. We've adapted that recipe to cut down on the preparation time and replaced the cipollini onions with easy-to-locate red onions.

SHOPPING LIST
6 medium red onions, peeled and quartered
1 cup balsamic vinegar
2 teaspoons honey
2 tablespoons olive oil
Salt, to taste

PREPARATION
Preheat an oven to 350°F. Place the quartered onions in a baking dish coated with olive oil. Season the onion with salt and bake for 20 minutes. Add the vinegar and honey, and cook for another 15-20 minutes, or until the onions have softened and the vinegar has reduced to a syrup-like consistency.

Prep time 5 minutes. *Total time* 40 minutes.

Serves 6.

Notes

Beans Baked with Tomatoes, Onions, and Molasses

With its high fiber and lycopene content from the tomato, this baked bean dish is surprisingly healthy for you. This simple recipe draws on a classic New England version of baked beans. We've used molasses instead of sugar due to its diverse nutrient profile, and replaced diced bacon with smoked pepper to avoid nitrates and pork fat.

SHOPPING LIST
1 32-ounce can butter beans
1 large onion, diced
1/4 cup molasses
3 ounces tomato paste
1 teaspoon Worcestershire sauce
1/2 teaspoon dry mustard
1 smoked pepper (optional)
Salt, to taste

PREPARATION
Sauté the onions until translucent. Rinse and drain the beans, then mix them with the molasses, Worcestershire sauce, ketchup, mustard, onions, and smoked pepper in a baking dish. Cover and cook at 350⁰ F for 45 minutes. Remove the smoked pepper before serving.

Prep time 1 hour.

Serves 4-6.

Notes

Roasted Tomato Casserole

Roasting tomatoes concentrates their flavor and releases lycopene. The following recipe pairs ripe tomatoes with fresh herbs, onions, and savory breadcrumbs. Try pairing this casserole with our Wine and Herb Poached Chicken.

SHOPPING LIST
Dressing
4 garlic cloves, minced
2 tablespoons balsamic vinegar
2 teaspoons Dijon mustard
3 tablespoons olive oil
1/2 teaspoon salt
1/4 teaspoon ground pepper
1/4 cup olive oil

Casserole
3 medium onions, sliced in thin rings
2 ½ pounds (about 8 to 10) large tomatoes, sliced into ½ inch slices
3/4 cup chopped fresh basil
2½ tablespoons fresh oregano, chopped
½ cup fresh parsley, chopped
3 tablespoons bread crumbs
3 tablespoons freshly grated Romano cheese (optional)
Salt, to taste

Garnish
1/4 cup basil leaves, torn

PREPARATION
Preheat the oven to 375°F. Combine all the dressing ingredients in a closed bottle and shake to mix. Arrange half of the onions in a baking dish and drizzle 1 tablespoon of the dressing

over the slices. Season with salt and pepper. Place half of the tomatoes over the onions, season with salt and pepper, and add another tablespoon of the dressing. Combine the herbs and sprinkle about half of the total herb amount on the tomatoes. Repeat with another layer of the onions, dressing, tomatoes, and herbs, making sure to season each layer with a little salt and pepper. Drizzle the remaining dressing on top of the casserole. Combine the breadcrumbs and cheese and sprinkle this mixture over the tomatoes. Bake the casserole for 1 hour. If the tomatoes are too juicy, pour off the excess liquid before serving.

Prep time 1-1/2 hours.

Serves 6.

Notes

Breakfast

Frittata

Traditionally, what grows now in the garden and what remains in the refrigerator from yesterday's dinner becomes frittata filling. We've offered a basic recipe with a list of possibilities for you to choose from, but the variations are endless. We build our frittatas by first wandering in our garden, picking copious herbs and vegetables, and then raiding our refrigerators to see what leftovers need to be used.

SHOPPING LIST
8-10 ounces egg whites
1/2 cup skim, soy, or rice milk
1 tablespoon olive oil
Salt and pepper, to taste

Filling
1/2 cup grated or crumbled nonfat cheese
1 cup vegetables, sliced or chopped (Onions, garlic, artichokes, asparagus, potatoes, mushrooms, spinach, kale, broccoli, carrots, zucchini, red or green peppers, or tomatoes)
2 tablespoons fresh herbs (Oregano, rosemary, basil, tarragon, chive, dill, or parsley)
1/2 cup leftover pasta, grains, or rice

PREPARATION
Place a rack in the upper third of the oven and preheat the oven to 350°F. Lightly beat the egg whites. Dampen a paper towel in olive oil and lightly grease an ovenproof skillet. Heat over medium high heat. Put the filling of your choice into the pan (cook the vegetables first if they are raw) then pour the eggs over the filling. Stir lightly until the eggs start to set. Reduce the heat to medium low. Once the bottom is firm and about one half inch thick, use a spatula to lift the edge of the frittata. Tilt the pan toward you so the uncooked egg

runs underneath. Lower the edge and swirl to distribute the egg. Continue cooking until the top is no longer runny. Put the skillet into the oven until the top is set and the inside just cooked through. Be careful not to overcook, because the eggs will be tough. Loosen the edges underneath the frittata and slide on to a serving plate. Season with salt and pepper. Serve hot, at room temperature, or chilled.

Prep time 30 minutes.

Serves 4.

Notes

Poached Egg Whites With Pesto and Greens

A quick nonfat way to cook, poaching allows egg whites to remain soft and delicate throughout the cooking process. While we love runny egg yolks, when we poach our whites we really don't miss the texture or flavor of the yolk. Below, we've provided a basic recipe for poaching one portion of whites (2 whites per portion). The basic formula is straightforward: for every gallon of salted water, add one teaspoon of vinegar to help the egg white cohere. Most cooks use distilled vinegar, but because of its neutral flavor we like using champagne or rice vinegar because of the trace of sweetness it adds to the dish. If you want to poach more eggs, simply use a larger pot/saucepan and more water/vinegar, and make sure the pot/saucepan has a wide mouth to make it easier to fetch the eggs. The pesto recipe mentioned is detailed in the Sauce section of this book. You can pair any vegetable you desire with this combination, but we recommend sautéing spinach in a separate pan with a little garlic, or following the Basic Greens recipe listed in the Side Dish section.

SHOPPING LIST
1 quart salt water
1/4 teaspoon vinegar, distilled, rice, or champagne
2 egg whites (do not beat)
Black pepper (optional and to taste)

PREPARATION
In a wide saucepan or shallow pot, place the salted water and vinegar. Bring the water to a low boil, reduce to a low simmer, and add the egg whites. Watch the eggs and the water: you do not want the water to cast bubbles; too much agitation will break apart the egg, and you want it to remain as whole as possible. Once the eggs are set, gently lift them from their hot water bath with a slotted spoon or metal spider. If you plan

on serving the eggs right away, pat the slotted spoon with a paper towel or serving napkin, and serve. If you plan on serving the whites later, cast them into a salted coldwater bath to stop the cooking process. Always pat the whites to make sure excess water does not cling to the surface. You may find the whites need additional salt and pepper, so be sure to check for seasoning before serving.

Prep time 10 minutes.

Serves 1-2.

Notes

Oatmeal with Seasonal Variations

Sometimes locating an oatmeal brand with quality flavorings becomes as challenging as finding a heart-healthy dish at a Super Bowl party. Below we've offered a list of ingredients you can use to dress up plain oatmeal. Our hope is that you won't rely on prepackaged oatmeal loaded with sugar and fillers, but add quality organic ingredients to plain oatmeal for better health and taste.

SHOPPING LIST
1 cup rolled oats
1 cup apple juice
1 cup water
Salt, to taste

Additions
1 tablespoon dried cranberries, or raisins
1/2 cup fresh or frozen strawberries, raspberries, blueberries, or banana
1 teaspoon ginger, grated
1/2 cinnamon
1 tablespoon honey, brown sugar, molasses, jam, or marmalade

PREPARATION
In a medium pot, bring the apple juice and water to a boil, season with a pinch of salt, and add the oatmeal. When the oatmeal is cooked halfway through, add your choice of dried, fresh, or frozen fruit, and finish the oatmeal. Remove from the heat, and stir in your choice of sweetener.

For quick oats, bring the apple juice and water to a boil, season with a pinch of salt, and add your choice of dried, fresh, or frozen fruit. Cook the fruit for 2-5 minutes, and add the oatmeal. Bring the mixture to a brief boil, and remove from the heat. Stir in your choice of honey, brown sugar, molasses, or fruit spread.

If you prefer to microwave your oatmeal: Combine the oats, liquids, and your choice of sweeteners and fruits in a large Pyrex bowl. Cook in the microwave on highest power for 3-5 minutes. Stir and serve.

Prep time 10 minutes.

Serves 2-4.

Notes

French Toast

Many breakfast dishes made with whole eggs, butter, and cream can be made without those ingredients. While we cannot make a biscuit worth its weight without butter, French toast made with egg whites and skim milk and lightly toasted in almond oil do taste better than the version fried in 1/2 pound of butter with 100% of your weekly cholesterol intake in egg yolk and cream. In many markets, you can even find free-range uncured unsmoked organic chicken links to pair with this crispy toast, but we like our French toast best with fresh blackberries, raspberries, or sliced peaches and a drizzle of honey.

SHOPPING LIST
6-8 ounces egg whites
2 tablespoons skim milk
1/2 teaspoon cinnamon
1/8 teaspoon nutmeg
Salt, to taste
8 slices whole wheat bread
1 tablespoon maple syrup or honey
1 tablespoon light olive oil or almond oil for toasting

PREPARATION
Put the whites in a shallow bowl, add the skim milk, cinnamon, and salt, and whisk until all the ingredients are incorporated. Dip the bread into the egg mixture and coat well on both sides. Brown the bread on both sides in a hot oiled skillet. Spread the toast on a platter, drizzle with warm syrup, honey, or fresh fruit.

Prep time 15 minutes

Serves 4.

Notes

Blueberry Pancakes

On special Sundays in the 1980s, we would make a delicious blueberry sauce for pancakes. We could smell the sweet cooked berry aroma drift through our house in the morning breeze, wafting into the living room where we all sat reading our favorite sections of the newspaper. You can substitute blackberries, strawberries, or raspberries for the blue. If you like more sweetness in your sauce, feel free to add honey or sugar to the mixture as it cooks.

SHOPPING LIST
Blueberry sauce
2 cups fresh or frozen blueberries
1 cup white grape juice or apple juice
2 tablespoons cornstarch or arrowroot

Pancakes
1-1/2 cups whole-wheat flour
1 tablespoon sugar
1-1/2 teaspoons baking powder
3/4 teaspoon baking soda
2 large egg whites
1-1/2 cups nonfat buttermilk or plain nonfat yogurt
1 teaspoon vanilla extract
1 cup blueberries

PREPARATION
Sauce
In a saucepan heat the berries and juice over low heat. Cook the berries until they begin to soften. Add the cornstarch, which you have premixed with a tablespoon of water. Stir the berry mixture until thickened.

Pancakes

In a large bowl mix, the flour, sugar, baking soda and baking powder. In a separate bowl mix together the egg whites, buttermilk or yogurt, and vanilla. Whisk the wet ingredients into the dry until smooth. Stir in the blueberries. Heat a griddle or skillet to medium high, coat it with light olive oil or almond oil, and drop the pancake batter ¼ cup at a time. Cook the cakes until bubbles form on the surface, flip, and cook the other side. Serve with the blueberry sauce and a sprinkle of powdered sugar.

Prep time 30 minutes

Serves 4.

Notes

Almond, Sunflower, and Raisin Muesli

Easy to assemble once you have the ingredients, muesli offers you a chance to control the amount of sugar, salt, and fat in your morning cereal. For this recipe, we like to visit the bulk bins and buy organic ingredients if they are available. You can substitute the almonds for pistachios, cashews, or pine nuts. Any dried fruit works in place of the raisins; if you use apricots, mango, apple, or pineapple, give the fruit a rough chop before adding it to the mix. Try muesli over nonfat yogurt or soymilk for a balanced and healthy breakfast.

SHOPPING LIST
1/2 cup almonds, ground
1 cup coconut, shredded
4 cups oats
1-1/2 cups raisins (or cranberries or blueberries)
1/2 cup sunflower seeds
1/8 cup powdered sugar, molasses, or honey
Pinch of salt, to taste
2 tablespoons olive oil, or almond oil

PREPARATION
Preheat an oven to 325°F. Mix the dry ingredients in a large baking dish. Drizzle the olive oil evenly over the surface of the dry ingredients, and then work in the olive oil. Bake the muesli for 45-60 minutes, or until toasted and brown. Stir the mixture every 5-10 minutes to ensure adequate toasting.

Prep Time 5 minutes

Serves 6-10

Notes

High-Rise Waffles

Waffles cooked in almond oil or olive oil and made with nonfat buttermilk allow you to enjoy the breakfast classic without breaking your healthy approach to diet.

SHOPPING LIST
1 cup whole wheat flour
1/8 teaspoon salt
1 teaspoon baking soda
1 large egg, separated
2 egg whites
1/4 cup nonfat buttermilk

PREPARATION
Plug in the waffle iron. Sift the flour, salt, and baking soda together in a large mixing bowl. In a separate bowl, lightly beat together the egg yolk and buttermilk, and stir the wet into the dry ingredients. Whip the egg whites until soft peaks form. Thoroughly fold the whites into the batter. Dab a hot waffle iron with almond oil or a light olive oil. Pour batter into the center of the waffle iron and cook until the indicator light goes out. Try topping these crispy waffles with our blueberry sauce mentioned earlier in this chapter.

Prep time 35 minutes.

Serves 4.

Notes

Egg White Omelet with Summer Vegetables

The following recipe provides basic instructions on how to make an egg white omelet. We've suggested using summer vegetables in this recipe, but feel free to substitute this list with whichever ripe and tasty vegetables you can find. In the spring, we love making omelets with asparagus, spring onion, and green garlic. In the winter, we use broccoli, cauliflower, or kale sautéed with caramelized onions to fill the omelets. The key to making this dish delicious rests in choosing the freshest vegetables and eggs you can find.

SHOPPING LIST
1 tablespoon olive oil
4 ounces egg whites
1 ounce soy, rice, or skim milk
1/2 cup mixture of onions, tomatoes, peppers, small diced
1 tablespoon mixed fresh oregano, basil, or parsley, chopped
Salt and pepper, to taste

Optional
1/2 cup nonfat cheese, soy, or rice cheese

PREPARATION
In a medium skillet, slowly caramelize the onions. Once the onions brown, add the peppers and tomatoes, season the vegetables with salt, and add the mixed chopped herbs. When they are just cooked through, scrap the vegetables onto a plate. In a shallow bowl, whisk the egg whites and milk, and season the mixture with salt and pepper. Slowly pour the egg mixture into the skillet and reduce the heat. Once the bottom of the omelet forms, lift an edge and let the uncooked liquid egg seep underneath. Add the vegetables and then the cheese. Cover the pan for 1-1/2 minutes. Once the surface of the omelet just sets,

fold the omelet and slide it onto a serving dish. Garnish with a sprinkle of fresh chopped herbs.

Prep time 12 minutes.

Serves 2.

Notes

Cherry and Pistachio Bran Muffins

Cherries and pistachios complement each other with their distinct flavors. We've combined them in these antioxidant and fiber packed muffins to allow you to eat a healthy breakfast on the go. Make a batch of muffins Sunday afternoon and during the week you will have a decent breakfast to snack on while you commute to work or rush to the gym.

SHOPPING LIST
1 cup whole-wheat flour
1 teaspoon baking soda
1/4 teaspoon salt
1-1/2 cups bran
2 tablespoons apple butter
1 tablespoon brown sugar
2 tablespoons molasses
1/4 cup egg whites
1-1/2 cups non-fat buttermilk
1/2 cup pistachios, chopped
1/2 cup dried cherries

PREPARATION
Preheated an oven to 375°F. Sift the flour, baking soda, and salt together. Stir the bran into the dry mixture. Beat together the apple butter, sugar and molasses, then add the mixed whites and buttermilk. Mix the dry and wet ingredients, and add the dried fruit and nuts. Fill paper muffin cups 1/2 full and bake the muffins for 15 to 20 minutes.

Prep time 15 minutes.

Serves 12 muffins.

Notes

Dessert

Decadent Chocolate Cake

Rich as it melts in your mouth, this chocolate cake is a good option for those on a low cholesterol diet. The Silken tofu provides a smooth texture and keeps the cake moist without the high cholesterol in eggs. It might come as a surprise that this cake is a great source of vegan protein! First make the frosting. Set aside to chill in the fridge until the cake is baked and cooled.

SHOPPING LIST

Frosting
1-1/2 cups sweetened vegan chocolate chips or baking chocolate
1/2 cup agave nectar
2 tablespoons light olive oil
12 ounce firm Silken tofu
1 cup unsweetened cocoa powder
1 teaspoon vanilla extract
1-3 teaspoons vanilla soymilk, as needed, to make the frosting creamy

Cake
1 cup all-purpose flour
1-1/2 teaspoon baking soda
1-1/2 teaspoon baking powder
3/4 teaspoon kosher salt
1 teaspoon vanilla
3/4 cups agave nectar
1-1/4 cups vegan chocolate chips or baking chocolate
12 ounces Silken tofu, cut in large chunks
1 cups cocoa powder

PREPARATION
Melt chocolate chips in a double boiler on low heat, stirring constantly until just melted. Place the chocolate, agave nectar,

olive oil, and tofu in a bowl and beat on high with a mixer until smooth and creamy. Beat in cocoa powder gradually until you reach the desired stiffness (so it won't run down sides of cake). If icing is too stiff, add a little soymilk. Chill the frosting in the refrigerator until the cake has cooled and you're ready to ice it.

Preheat oven to 350°F. Oil two 8" round cake pans. Place a pan on a sheet of wax paper and trace it with a pen. Cut out two circles and place them in the pans. Melt the chocolate chips in a double boiler on low heat, again stirring continually until just melted, and set aside. Combine flour, baking soda, baking powder, and salt in a bowl. Use a nonstick spatula to mix well and set aside. Place melted chocolate, tofu, cocoa powder, agave nectar, and vanilla in a food processor. Process until smooth. Pour chocolate mixture into dry ingredients and mix well. Spread evenly into the pans using your nonstick spatula. Bake for 20-25 minutes or until a tooth-pick placed in the center comes out clean. (For a 9 x12 sheet pan, approximately 35 minutes.) Remove from pans and cool on racks. Frost when the cake has cooled.

Stuffed Baked Apples

Apples baked with cinnamon will fill your house with the aromas of baked apple pie, but this dish skips the butter and flour crust and replaces it with plumped dried fruit and a refreshing spoonful of yogurt. Feel free to substitute the apples with baked pears.

SHOPPING LIST
4 medium baking apples
1/4 cup raisins
1/4 cup dried cranberries
2 tablespoons honey
1 tablespoon brown sugar
1 cup apple juice
1/2 teaspoon cinnamon, ground
4 ounces nonfat vanilla yogurt
Salt, to taste

PREPARATION
Preheat an oven to 350°F. Wash, peel, and partially core the apples. In a small bowl combine the dried fruits, brown sugar, honey, and 2 tablespoons of apple juice. Stuff the apple cavities with the fruit mixture. Pour the remaining apple juice into a baking dish and place the apples in it. Cover the baking dish and bake the apples for 30-40 minutes. Remove the dish from the oven when the apples are cooked through. Garnish each apple with a dab of yogurt and a sprinkle of cinnamon.

Prep time 1 hour.

Serves 4.

Notes

Seasonal Berries with Yogurt and Mint

Fresh berries straight from the farmers' market or culled from your backyard garden create a simple and healthy dessert. This basic recipe will work well with any berries you can find—try variations that include blackberries and currants.

SHOPPING LIST
1 cup fresh or frozen raspberries
1 cup fresh or frozen strawberries
1 cup fresh or frozen blueberries
1 tablespoon sugar
1 teaspoon lemon zest
1 tablespoon lemon juice
Salt, to taste

Optional Garnish
4 mint sprigs
4 tablespoons nonfat yogurt

PREPARATION
For fresh berries clean, wash, and drain the berries of water. For frozen berries, partially thaw, wash, and drain the berries of water. In a large bowl, place the berries, lemon zest, lemon juice, and sugar. Stir the mixture to make sure the ingredients evenly coat the berries. Let the mixture stand for one hour. Serve the berry mixture in small bowls, and garnish with fresh mint leaves and nonfat yogurt. Another serving option is to spoon the berry mixture over Angel food cake. Angel food cake is made without butter and egg yolks, so it is a safer dessert for you to pair with these berries than shortcakes or pastry dough.

Prep time 10-15 minutes. *Total time* 1-1/4 hours.

Serves 8.

Tangy Peach Crisp

Crisps traditionally contain buttered toppings, which help create the characteristic crunch and rich flavor the dessert is known for. We've dropped the butter from our recipe, and think that the topping does not need any dairy fat to help it crisp. Feel free to substitute any fruit for the peaches.

SHOPPING LIST
8 cups fresh peaches, sliced
3 tablespoons tapioca
1/2 cup pineapple juice
2 tablespoons honey
1 teaspoon cinnamon
1/8 teaspoon salt

Crisp topping
1 1/3 cups rolled oats
1/2 cup whole-wheat flour
1/4 cup oat flour
2 tablespoons honey
1/4 cup orange juice
1 teaspoon vanilla extract
1/2 teaspoon olive oil
Salt, to taste

PREPARATION
Preheat oven to 375°F. Soften the tapioca in pineapple juice in a small bowl for 5 minutes. Mix the tapioca into the remaining wet ingredients. Place the peach mixture into a baking dish lightly oiled with a neutral or light olive oil and bake for 15-20 minutes. In the meantime, make the crisp topping. Combine the dry ingredients and the wet (honey, orange juice, vanilla) ingredients separately. Pour the liquid ingredients over the dry and stir until mixed. Take the baked peaches out of the oven,

stir, and crumble the topping evenly over the peaches. Bake the dish for another 20 minutes, or until the topping becomes crisp.

Prep time 1-1/4 hours.

Serves 6.

Carrot Cake with Dried Fruits

SHOPPING LIST
1 cup carrots, grated
1/4 cup dates, chopped
1/2 cup raisins
1/2 cup dried cranberries, chopped
1 1/3 cups white wine or apple juice
1/4 cup applesauce
1 teaspoon cinnamon
1/8 teaspoon cloves, ground
1/8 teaspoon nutmeg, ground
1 teaspoon baking powder
1 teaspoon baking soda
2 cups whole wheat flour
1/8 teaspoon salt

Icing
1 cup nonfat plain yogurt
1/2 teaspoon vanilla extract
1 tablespoon sugar
1/8 teaspoon salt

PREPARATION
Preheat the oven to 350°F. In a saucepan simmer the dried fruits, white wine, applesauce, and warm spices for 5 minutes, or until the dried fruits plump and the mixture reduces into a loose sauce. Cool. Mix the dry ingredients together (including the carrot), then combine wet with the dry ingredients and stir until well blended. Spoon the batter into an 8" x 8" oiled cake pan and bake for 45 minutes. Un-mold the cake onto a large plate. You may need to run a knife along the cake to loosen it from the pan. Allow the cake to cool. Make the icing by combing the yogurt, vanilla extract, sugar, and salt in a large bowl. Whisk the ingredients

until smooth, about one minute. Once the cake has cooled completely, drizzle the icing over the cake and serve.

Prep time 1 hour.

Serves 4-8.

Notes

Rice Pudding With Almonds and Golden Raisins

Sweetened with honey and flavored with vanilla and cinnamon, rice pudding becomes a healthy dessert when you substitute skim, soy, or rice milk for heavy cream.

SHOPPING LIST
4 cups brown rice, cooked
2 cups soy, rice or skim milk
1/2 cup golden raisins
1/2 cup almonds, roasted and chopped fine
3 tablespoons honey
1 teaspoon cinnamon
1 teaspoon vanilla extract

PREPARATION
Preheat oven to 325°F. In a saucepan, combine all the ingredients and stir constantly for 15-20 minutes, or until creamy, hot, and slightly bubbling. Sprinkle with cinnamon. Can be served hot or cold.

Prep time 5 minutes. *Total time* 55 minutes.

Serves 4.

Notes

Spicy Ginger Snaps

Ginger snaps made from a mixture of warm spices will help kick your digestive system into gear. This recipe contains no dairy fat, so you can feel virtuous while you eat snap after snap.

SHOPPING LIST
2-1/2 cups all-purpose flour
2 teaspoons baking soda
3 teaspoons ginger, ground
1 teaspoon cinnamon, ground
1 teaspoon dry mustard
1/2 teaspoon white pepper
1/8 teaspoon cardamom, ground
1/8 teaspoon cloves, ground
1/4 teaspoon salt
3/4 cup apple butter
1 cup dark brown sugar, packed
2 ounces egg whites
1/4 cup molasses
3 tablespoons granulated sugar

PREPARATION
Preheat the oven to 350°F. In a large bowl, mix all of the dry ingredients except the sugars. In a mixer on medium speed, whisk the apple butter and brown sugar until blended. Add the molasses and egg and mix until combined. Reduce the speed to low and continue to mix for one minute. While still on low speed, add the dry ingredients. Once the dust settles, turn the speed up until the dry ingredients are completely incorporated. Divide the dough in half, shape each half into a ball, and pat each ball flat into a puck. Wrap each puck with wax paper or plastic wrap, and refrigerate for 1-2 hours. Shape the dough into 1-inch balls, roll each ball in granulated sugar, and set each cookie at least 2 inches apart on a parchment-lined or nonstick

cookie sheet. Bake the snaps until brown on the bottom, about 5 minutes. Rotate the sheet to ensure even baking and cook another 5 minutes. Cool the snaps on the sheet for 5 minutes, and then place them on a rack while they continue to cool. Eat the cookies immediately, or store them in an airtight container.

Prep time 30 minutes to prepare and bake, plus the time to cool the mixture.

Serves 36 cookies.

Notes

Oatmeal Drop Cookies

Many cookie recipes list butter as the main ingredient, but unlike croissant dough or puff pastry, cookies do not need butter for their unique texture or flavor. Oatmeal drop cookies have the added benefit of high fiber content from oats, raisins, and nuts.

SHOPPING LIST
1/2 cup olive oil
3/4 cup granulated sugar
1/4 cup egg whites, lightly whisked
1-1/2 cup unbleached flour
1/2 teaspoon salt
1/2 teaspoon baking soda
3/4 teaspoon cinnamon, ground
1/8 teaspoon cloves, ground
1/8 teaspoon allspice, ground
1-3/4 cups rolled oats
2/3 cups raisins, chopped
1/2 cup chopped almonds, pistachios, or cashews
1/3 cup non-fat skim milk

PREPARATION
Preheat the oven to 350°F. In a large bowl mix the oil and sugar, and then beat in whisked egg whites. Add the flour and spices, and mix all the ingredients until smooth. Add the raisins and nuts alternately with the milk. Using a tablespoon, drop the dough onto oiled cookie sheets. Bake for about 15 minutes, or until the cookies are set in the middle and brown on the edges.

Prep time 15 minutes. *Total time* 30 minutes.

Serves 4.

Raspberry Custard

The following recipe allows you to enjoy the delicate texture of custard without the cream and egg yolks. When blended, Silken tofu makes a smooth and protein-packed alternative to traditional custards. Any combination of raspberries, blueberries, blackberries, and huckleberries can substitute for the berries listed in this recipe.

SHOPPING LIST
14 ounces Silken tofu
6 ounces fresh or frozen raspberries
2 ounces fresh or frozen strawberries
1/2 teaspoon vanilla extract
2 tablespoons sugar

PREPARATION
In a blender, mix the tofu and strawberries; add the sugar and vanilla and blend until smooth. Pour the mixture into custard cups and refrigerate for at least an hour. Garnish with fresh raspberries or diced strawberries.

Prep time 15 minutes. *Total time* 1-1/4 hours.

Serves 4.

Notes

Almond and Coconut Date Rolls

Date rolls taste like rich candy, but contain no dairy fat. This recipe is easy to follow and takes no time to execute. We often substitute pistachios or pine nuts for the almonds, and encourage you to try each variation.

SHOPPING LIST
1/2 cup almonds, toasted and finely chopped
1/2 coconut, shredded
1/8 cup powdered sugar (optional)
2-3 tablespoons honey
1/8 teaspoon salt
12 pitted Medjool dates

PREPARATION
In a wide bowl, mix the almonds, coconut, and powdered sugar. Roll each date in honey until lightly coated, and place it in the bowl. Pack the date with the almond/coconut mixture until it adheres to the sides of the date. Place the dates on a plate lined with wax paper until ready to serve.

Prep Time 10 minutes.

Serves 6-12.

Notes

Ossi di Morti

Ossi di Morti means "bones of the dead" in Italian. These delicate cookies are prepared as treats for All Souls' Day on November 2nd. Skilled bakers often spread the cookies out to resemble skeletons before baking. Try these slightly sweet cookies with a cup of coffee for a nice afternoon treat.

SHOPPING LIST
3/4 cup sugar
1/3 cup flour
3/4 teaspoon baking powder
2 egg whites
1-1/4 cups almonds, lightly toasted and roughly chopped
1/2 teaspoon almond extract
Pinch of salt
1/2 teaspoon cinnamon for sprinkling on the cooled cookies

PREPARATION
Preheat an oven to 325°F. In a large bowl, mix together the sugar, flour, and baking powder. Add the beaten egg whites and mix until the whites and dry ingredients combine. Stir in the almonds until combined. In a parchment-lined and oiled sheet tray, drop one tablespoon per cookie. Make sure to allow 2"-3" around each cookie. If you feel festive, with a spatula gently spread out each cookie to resemble a bone. Bake the cookies for 15-18 minutes, or until golden brown. (Don't forget to rotate the sheet trays to ensure even cooking.) Remove the tray from the oven and allow the cookies to cool before removing and sprinkling with cinnamon.

Prep Time 20-30 minutes.

Serves 20 cookies

Lemon Granita

Granita can refresh you on a hot summer day, or help cleanse your palate in-between courses. You can make this dish ahead of time, but be sure to temper the granita by bringing it out of the freezer to loosen. We prefer to top our granita with a drizzle of the strawberry sauce listed, but the strong lemon in this granita can stand on its own as well.

SHOPPING LIST
1 cup lemon juice
1 cup sugar
1 cup water
1 tablespoon lemon zest

Strawberry Sauce
2 cups strawberries, cut in half
1/3 cup water (if using fresh berries)
1 teaspoon sugar
1/2 inch strip of lemon peel
Pinch of salt

PREPARATION
In a medium saucepan, mix the sugar and water. Heat and stir the liquid until the sugar dissolves. Remove the pan from the heat, pour the sugar water into a freezer-proof baking dish, and let the mixture cool. Stir in the lemon juice and zest, and place the dish in the freezer. Stir the granita every hour to half hour for six hours, or until the granita sets completely; you are looking for a slushy-like consistency. Serve lemon granita in a cold glass or dish, and drizzle the top with fresh strawberry sauce.

Strawberry sauce

In a medium saucepan, place the strawberries, lemon peel, salt, and water. Cover the pan 3/4 of the way to allow steam to escape, and cook the berries on very low heat until they soften completely. Taste the berries to see if they need sugar, and then allow the mixture to cool to room temperature. Puree the sauce until smooth. Place it in the refrigerator to cool before serving.

Prep Time 20 minutes. *Total Time* 4-6 hours for granita to set.

Serves 4-5

Notes

Beverages

Green Tea

We have found that green tea can be rather bland, but if you add honey, ginger, and lemon you can turn it into a delicious and revitalizing drink.

SHOPPING LIST
Green tea
Sugar or honey
Ginger
Lemon

PREPARATION
While boiling the water put the tea and grated ginger into a tea ball. Place the tea ball into a teapot. Pour the boiling water into the teapot. Let the tea steep for 5-8 minutes. Remove the ball, and add lemon and honey to taste. Serve the tea hot or cold. We often make large quantities and refrigerate for a refreshing iced beverage.

Prep time 15 minutes.

Serves Various.

Notes

Berry Shake

If you crave a milkshake, but don't dare risk the fat, try this recipe to sooth your craving. We use frozen berries for this recipe because they remind us of the texture that ice cream gives to a milkshake. You can use mixed berries or concentrate on a single berry.

SHOPPING LIST
1/2 pound Silken tofu
1 cup frozen mixed berries (or 1 cup single berry of your choosing)
1 teaspoon vanilla extract
1 cup skim, soy, or rice milk
Sugar or sweetener, to taste

PREPARATION
In a blender, blend the milk and tofu. Add the berries and vanilla and continue to blend for 1 ½ minutes, or until the mixture is smooth and all ingredients have blended together. Pour into two chilled tall glasses and serve.

Prep time 10 minutes.

Serves 2.

Notes

Healthy Holiday Eggnog

You can enjoy eggnog's richness without the excessive fat that accompanies the original version. This recipe allows you to engage in a holiday tradition without sacrificing your health. It does have alcohol, but is virtually fat free.

SHOPPING LIST
8 ounces Eggbeaters
3 tablespoons sugar
1 quart skim, soy, or rice milk
1 pint dark rum
4 ounces bourbon
1 pint non-fat frozen vanilla yogurt
1 teaspoon cinnamon
1 teaspoon freshly grated nutmeg

PREPARATION
In a food processor or blender, mix the Eggbeaters and sugar. Gradually add half the milk, all of the bourbon, and all of the rum. Let stand for 10 minutes, then add the remaining milk, frozen yogurt, and cinnamon. Serve in a pretty punch bowl, sprinkled with nutmeg.

Prep time 25 minutes.

Serves 10-12.

Notes

Hot Spiced Cider

This drink is wonderful after a cold winter walk in the woods. We find that fresh-pressed cider, still cloudy with apple particles, provides the best flavor.

SHOPPING LIST
1 quart apple cider
2-3 cinnamon sticks
1 teaspoon freshly grated ginger
1/8 teaspoon nutmeg
1/8 teaspoon allspice

PREPARATION
Heat cider and add the spices, simmering for 10 minutes. Serve with a cinnamon stick.

Prep time 15 Minutes.

Serves 4.

Notes

Hot Chocolate

Hot chocolate on a snowy day can comfort and sooth every muscle in your body. This version pairs antioxidant-rich chocolate with skim milk for healthy nourishment without dangerous dairy fat. Note that the chocolate must be pure chocolate and contain no dairy fat.

SHOPPING LIST
1 quart skim, soy, or rice milk
1/4 cup powdered unsweetened cocoa
1/3 cup water
1/4 cup sugar
1/4 cup grated dark unsweetened chocolate

PREPARATION
Slowly heat the water in a saucepan. Add the sugar and cocoa, and whisk the ingredients until incorporated. Stir in the skim milk. Continue to stir and heat the mixture until it comes to a low simmer. Serve in mugs with grated chocolate sprinkled on top.

Prep time 15 Minutes.

Serves 4.

Notes

Mulled Wine

One of our favorite holiday recipes, this mulled wine offers your guests a festive drink with little preparation. Oranges and lemons contain antioxidant properties, and cinnamon adds additional health benefits.

SHOPPING LIST
2 cups water
1/2 cup honey
2 cloves
3 sticks cinnamon
2 lemons, thinly sliced
1 orange, thinly sliced
1 bottle red wine
3 ounces brandy

PREPARATION
Bring the water to a boil, reduce the heat, and add the honey and spices. Simmer the liquid for five minutes. Add the lemons and let the liquid steep for 10 minutes. Add the wine and brandy and heat gently; do not boil. Put the oranges into a stainless steel or glass punch bowl (never put hot liquids in plastic containers) and add the mulled wine. Serve immediately.

Prep time 30 minutes.

Serves 8.

Notes

Stock

We prefer to make our own stock so that we can control the amount of fat and salt. We often make pure vegetable stocks, and occasionally a well skimmed chicken or fish stock. We do not use beef or pork.

Once the stock is made we freeze or store it in various-sized containers. A great trick is to freeze a substantial amount in ice cube trays and transfer them to freezer bags or containers. Freezing a variety of sizes allows you to use whatever you need without waste.

Basic rules for stock making:

Rinse all bones and vegetables throughly in cold running water.

Start by placing the vegetables or bones in the pot and adding the desired amount of cold water.

Do not add more than a pinch of salt to the stock base. If you add salt, by the time the stock reduces you might have an overseasoned batch of stock.

Skim the proteins and impurities that bubble to the surface of the stock with a shallow ladle and discard.

For a rich dark stock, try roasting your vegetables or bones in the oven before simmering.

Vegetable Stock

SHOPPING LIST
1 cup each of the following vegetables:
celery
onions
carrots
leeks
4 garlic cloves, smashed
5-8 parsley stems
5 whole peppercorns
1 bay leaf
1-1/2 gallons water

PREPARATION
Wash and slice the vegetables into inch-long pieces. Place the vegetables in a deep pot. Pour cold water into the pot. Slowly bring the mixture to a boil, and immediately reduce to a simmer. Cook for 1-1/2 to 2 hours. Strain all the vegetables for a clear stock. For a richer and darker stock, try roasting the vegetables in an oven at 375°F until slightly browned.

Prep time 15 minutes. *Total time* 2-1/4 hours.

Notes

Chicken Stock

SHOPPING LIST
Bones from one chicken
1 cup each of the following vegetables, chopped
celery
onion
leeks
carrots
5 garlic cloves, smashed
5 whole peppercorns
1 bay leaf
1–1-1/2 gallons of water

PREPARATION
Add the cold water to a large stockpot. Add the chicken bones, vegetables, bay leaf, and peppercorns, and bring the liquid to a boil. Reduce the liquid to a low simmer, and cook for two to four hours. Occasionally, use a spoon to skim the proteins that bubble to the surface. Strain the stock through a colander and into a new pot to remove the chicken bones and vegetables. Once your stock has cooled to room temperature, place the stock in the refrigerator until fat solidifies on the top. Take the stock from the refrigerator and carefully remove fat with a spoon.

Prep time 15 minutes. *Total time* 2–3-1/2 hours.

Notes

Fish Stock

Lean fish work best for a neutral and versatile stock that you can use as a soup or sauce base. We find halibut, cod, bass, and other white-fleshed fish bones work best for stocks. Fish such as salmon, sardines, and mackerel tend to be oily and have such a strong flavor that they will dominate other ingredients.

SHOPPING LIST
2 pounds fish bones (you can use heads and tails,
    as well as body parts)
1 cup each of the following vegetables, chopped
    celery
    onion
    leeks
1 bay leaf
2 quarts water
2 cups of white wine

PREPARATION
Pour 2 quarts of cold water and white wine into your pot. Add the fish parts, vegetables, and bay leaf and bring the liquid to a strong simmer. Do not boil the liquid as boiling will make a cloudy stock. Reduce the heat to a low simmer and cook for one and half to two hours. Occasionally, use a spoon to skim the proteins that bubble to the surface. Drain the stock through a colander to remove the fish bones and vegetables. Cool the liquid in the refrigerator until fat solidifies on the top. Take the stock from the refrigerator and carefully remove the fat.

Prep time 15 minutes. *Total time* 2-1/4 hours.

Notes